Digital Therapy

Technological Prospects and Social Applications Set

coordinated by
Bruno Salgues

Volume 6

Digital Therapy

The New Age of Healthcare

Laure Beyala

iSTE

WILEY

First published 2022 in Great Britain and the United States by ISTE Ltd and John Wiley & Sons, Inc.

ISTE Ltd
27-37 St George's Road
London SW19 4EU
UK

www.iste.co.uk

John Wiley & Sons, Inc.
111 River Street
Hoboken, NJ 07030
USA

www.wiley.com

Library of Congress Control Number: 2022943898

British Library Cataloguing-in-Publication Data
A CIP record for this book is available from the British Library
ISBN 978-1-78630-800-9

Introduction

France, Germany and Russia, along with most countries in the world, have been confronted at least once in their history with unprecedented phenomena involving increases in serious chronic pathologies that affected all sectors of activity.

The World Health Organization (WHO) defines chronic diseases as "any health problem that requires ongoing management over several years, usually resulting in long-stay hospital admissions and intensive care".

As a reminder, chronic diseases affect more than 30% of adults in developed countries, cause the premature death of more than 550,000 people of working age each year and account for more than 75% of healthcare spending in European countries.

According to the IMS-Health Continuous Prescription Survey (CPPS), between the ages of 25 and 64, the top three reasons for ambulatory care are, in almost equal proportions, cardiovascular disease, diseases of the respiratory system and diseases of the osteoarticular system.

Among those 65 years and older, osteoarthritis, lower back pain or other chronic back injury and high blood pressure are the most frequently reported conditions or health problems.

Today, patients with chronic diseases increasingly need care. However, most current health systems, developed to respond particularly to congenital[1], hereditary[2] or acute[3] diseases, are not always adapted to manage such health conditions.

In this sense, we can note the considerable emergence of new organizations in the medical field brought about by advances in information and communication technologies (ICT). One of these advances is represented the contribution of 5G, which has provided intelligent algorithms introducing new architectures and new services at all levels in the care of patients, including the prevention, diagnosis, treatment and monitoring of physiological health parameters.

Even if we recognize that these medical technologies disrupt existing organizational methods, specializations and services in the care strategy, it is important to emphasize that this new pace of technological innovation driven by ICT generates opportunities that embody the remarkable potential of digital therapy to significantly improve care through predictive, preventive, personalized, participatory, precision- and evidence-based medicine.

The prowess of medical innovations lies in the better management of healthcare structures, as well as in the reduction of costs related to the care of patients.

As can be seen during the follow-up of a patient with a chronic disease, healthcare professionals are increasingly encouraging individuals to adopt emerging digital technologies to address their health conditions.

What would be the drivers of the adoption of this digital therapy in our communities in the short, medium and long term?

In its first part, this scientific study gives an overview of the catalyzing societal context of new disruptive technologies in healthcare. Then, we present a comparative analysis of technological solutions that will

1 A disease or malformation present at birth. Congenital diseases can be due to genetic abnormalities, the intrauterine environment or unknown factors.

2 A disease transmitted to an individual in their genes. This disease, genetically inherited by the child, is transmitted by the parents. The disease can be dominant (i.e. occurring in each generation) or recessive (i.e. occurring from time to time).

3 Acute illness is an alteration in the general state of health. It is characterized by identified symptoms, progression and recovery.

exhibit remarkable growth in medicine in the coming year propelled by the needs expressed by populations duri epidemics and outbreaks of rare and severe diseases.

Finally, we study the mechanisms that need to be put in the adoption and democratization of digital health technology

PART 1

Medical Innovation

1

A Conceptual Framework for Health Innovations

1.1. Introduction

Innovation is undoubtedly the best strategy for confronting the challenges faced by the world of health. It is one way to meet the demand for health services without increasing the budgetary envelope of public funds allocated to the health field. It is imperative to increase efficiency. From this perspective, the only logical and realistic solution is the successful integration of innovations.

1.2. Defining innovation

An innovation can be a new thought or a new product perceived as useful by an individual or an organization because it brings a new answer to an encountered problem. It is a dynamic approach that leads to a solution that meets an identified need.

The innovation can have a physical form, with superior performances in terms of ergonomic aspects and the functionalities of use. It can also be entirely composed of information, such as a political vision or a business idea.

It should be noted that research[1], for its part, is a factor of great importance in innovation. Research refers to all the actions that promote increases in knowledge in relation to the state of the art in a particular field. Thus, we speak of technological innovation because it covers innovation derived from research.

Beyond the term "technological innovation" cited above, according to the Organisation for Economic Co-operation and Development (OECD) and the European Commission[2], there are other types of innovation, including product, process, marketing and organizational innovation:

– product innovations[3] can be defined as the development of a good that is significantly improved in terms of its characteristics or intended use; this assessment of innovation concerns significant improvements in technical specifications, components and materials, usability or other functional characteristics;

– process innovations can be defined as the implementation of a new or significantly improved production or distribution method;

– marketing innovations refer to the implementation of a new marketing method involving significant changes to the design, packaging or pricing of a particular product;

– organizational innovations consist of implementing a new organizational method in the practices, workplace organization or external relations of the company. They also involve can be the organization of finances or the workforce.

1.2.1. *Different levels of innovation*

Although the term "disruptive innovation" is most often attributed to new concepts from the medical field, the scientific literature emphasizes that there are other levels of innovation. Innovation can be incremental or radical. It can also be the end result of the development of new business ideas.

1 The French term "*recherche*" means "the action of searching, but in various fields it has a more precise or figurative meaning" (https://fr.wikipedia.org/wiki/Recherche).

2 Available at: https://www.oecd.org/site/innovationstrategy/defininginnovation.htm.

3 As defined in the Oslo Manual.

1.2.1.1. *Adjacent innovation*

Adjacent innovation is one of the most common strategies used to extend the life of a service or product. This form of innovation allows an existing product to be taken to another market for which it was not intended or the creation of a new product in an existing market.

1.2.1.2. *Radical innovation*

This form of innovation consists of commercializing a new product in a new market. This concept does not respond to the existing problems in a company since the innovative company will tackle a brand new market with its freshly created product. This type of innovation creates new uses and new paradigms.

1.2.1.3. *Disruptive innovation*

Disruptive innovation provides access to a particular service either by simplifying its use or reducing its price. This level of innovation allows for the rapid acquisition of market shares. It also makes it possible to considerably avoid disruption. For example, prices can be slashed by simplifying a product or process. Thus, disruptive innovation is the opposite of incremental innovation.

1.2.1.4. *Incremental innovation*

Incremental innovation corresponds to the improvement of an existing service or product. This initiative is put in place in order to offer something different without taking unnecessary risks. In this way, offerings can compete on the basis of better quality, lower prices and easier-to-use features for end users. Incremental innovation is the most accessible kind of innovation in our societies. Most of the time, the public already knows the product and does not need to be convinced of its added value.

1.2.1.5. *Examples of disruptive and incremental innovations in digital health*

1.2.1.5.1. Connected sphygmomanometers

The launch of the MyThermo connected blood pressure monitor as a connected medical device by the Visiomed Group represents a disruptive innovation. This class IIa blood pressure monitor is a CE-marked medical device. It is designed to monitor changes in arterial measurements. The data are sent immediately to a mobile terminal and are hosted by a certified health host. The device weighs 245 g and contains a microfiber pouch, a user guide, four AA alkaline batteries and a cuff.

The iHealth BP5 IHealth multioption connected blood pressure monitor, a connected medical device produced and marketed by the iHealth laboratory, represents an incremental innovation in terms of the weight of the device. Connected to a smartphone by Bluetooth, it works on the iHealth My Vitals application (iOS and Android) and weighs 135 g.

Withings BPM Connect is a medical device that measures blood pressure and heart rate with medical precision. This device synchronizes via Wi-Fi or Bluetooth. It works with a rechargeable battery that can be used for 6 months with a single charge. It is therefore an incremental innovation.

1.2.1.5.2. Case study: smart thermometers

The Withings Thermo smart temporal thermometer, marketed by the company Withings, transfers the data collected by the thermo application via a Wi-Fi network (iOS and Android). The net weight of the product is about 75 g. The medical accuracy is ±0.2°C for the display of values equivalent to a rectal temperature reading. This is a disruptive innovation.

The FT 95 infrared non-contact thermometer marketed by Beurer is a CE-marked medical device that measures body, ambient and surface temperature. It transfers the collected data via Bluetooth to the Beurer BabyCare application. The net weight of the product is approximately 73 g; it has a measuring distance of 2–3 cm and an accuracy of ±0.2°C between 34 and 42.2°C (±0.4°F: 93.2–108°F). This is an incremental innovation.

In view of the above examples, incremental innovation should be perceived as an iterative system where a product with small improvements is presented each time.

However, there are factors that can encourage the implementation of disruptive innovations in the health field. These are exogenous factors and endogenous factors. Exogenous factors can be linked to environmental, political and/or societal crises. Endogenous factors are related to regulations, organizational structures, business models and the expertise of providers working in the existing healthcare system.

Among the exogenous factors related to the living environment, we can identify environmental crises, which include pollution, the disruption of our aquatic ecosystem, climate change, epidemics and so on. They are real catalysts for the occurrence of chronic non-communicable diseases. Social factors include problems related to demographic crises.

1.2.2. *Endogenous factors of disruptive innovation in digital health*

1.2.2.1. *Organizational structure*

Most developed countries have opted for national health strategies specific to their historical, political and social contexts. Developing and low- and middle-income countries are also striving to achieve universal access to healthcare and health for all by expanding primary healthcare and social security schemes.

In France, in the Middle Ages, the Church was the main actor in the fight against growing poverty and held a monopoly on assistance. The first establishments for the most destitute were instituted under the name of "Hôtels-Dieu". Aid to the destitute began to be structured in the 13th century with the "tables of the poor". However, under the Ancien Régime, almsgiving and charity were municipalized and secularized, thus responding to the concern for maintaining public order.

In the medieval and Renaissance eras, guilds provided prepaid healthcare to members and their families.

Today, several approaches to national health insurance and national health services have been developed, such as the Bismarck social security model and the Beveridge national health system. The latter was developed in 1942 in the United Kingdom by Lord Beveridge. At the time, he considered the British compulsory health insurance system to be "too limited with the ceiling system, too complex with the multitude of funds and poorly coordinated". Many developed countries have several universal health insurance systems. It is worth recalling that Otto von Bismarck, the German chancellor, introduced the first health insurance system for workers. It is a social insurance system based on contributions, so benefits are given to those who have contributed.

1.2.2.2. *Influence of the political agenda*

However, the global architecture in the 20th century still abounded with multiple barriers and major gaps preventing the healthcare system in many states from meeting the physical and social needs of populations. This was reflected in barriers to access to primary care and ambulatory care, time constraints preventing the effective management of care center provision, a lack of attention to social factors and competing professional and personal obligations. Also present were high levels of morbidity in poorer populations, the spread of pandemics and epidemics, technological innovation, the high cost of both medical care and research and the high cost of health insurance.

Moreover, there is no common benchmark for universal access to healthcare in all countries of the world. Each country develops and adapts a national health program that corresponds to its own health needs. Every healthcare system is under pressure everywhere, not only to ensure access to healthcare for all citizens but also to keep up with the progress of medical technologies.

This architecture highlights the need to influence the political agenda in order to accelerate the development of disruptive innovations in the medical field, knowing that these technological innovations encompass the integration of new organizational processes within healthcare institutions, with the ultimate goal of improving healthcare and the operational efficiency of healthcare personnel.

The long wait times for treaetments in some healthcare facilities could be reduced by the increased adoption of technology through digital medical therapy, which would allow patients to monitor their health indicators at home and communicate this information to healthcare professionals remotely.

As a result, health systems in several countries are beginning to implement health reforms to promote equity, efficiency and digital technologies to ensure access to quality care for populations of all socioeconomic statuses. These reforms most often include the development of stable health institutions, best practice approaches to governance and policy-relevant budgeting strategies.

1.2.3. *Exogenous factors of disruptive innovation in digital health*

As a variable that facilitates the implementation of an innovation, a reform certainly cannot achieve its final objective if it does not take into account other exogenous factors.

These factors could be related to the demographic, environmental and social crises in our communities.

1.2.3.1. *Demographic crises*

Changing demographics are fundamental to public health and healthcare services, as the composition of the population determines the volume and nature of the health needs to be adapted to address a particular threat.

Based on patients' environmental context, several types of needs can be distinguished in the current care setting:

– needs requiring technological devices focused on the patient or the general public: these are devices related to e-health whose services revolve around mobile health applications, connected health objects, social networks for health professionals, teaching and patient monitoring platforms;

– needs requiring technological devices focused on care providers, such as health institutions and health professionals – for instance, telemedicine devices;

– needs requiring technological devices focused on insurance, public regulators and industrial players. These include generic customer relationship management tools (CRM), as well as data mining tools (internal data) and Big Data (external data) enabling the collection, hosting and algorithmic processing of massive health data.

In the next section, we focus on older populations.

1.2.3.1.1. An ageing population

The beginning of the 21st century was marked by an exponential increase in the ageing of the population. It is worth noting that in some countries, particularly in sub-Saharan Africa, there is a demographic explosion among young people. In most nations, existing health systems are struggling to

existing healthcare institutions. It requires a reorganization of care delivery to maintain interactions between caregivers and patients.

– The development and adoption of such technologies could also foster the creation of new business models to support the deployment of digital therapy for the elderly.

– The creation and reinforcement of cooperation networks between public and private sector providers and learned societies in order to allow access to remote care for the elderly and frail.

1.2.3.2. *Environmental crises*

1.2.3.2.1. Degradation of aquatic ecosystems

An aquatic ecosystem is an ecosystem[4] in and surrounding a body of water, especially fresh water. A marine aquatic ecosystem can be constituted by lagoons, mangroves, lagoon areas (brackish water), etc. In a freshwater environment, an aquatic ecosystem is the result of a balance between a natural habitat and all of the animal and plant species that live there.

In good health, this ecosystem provides essential goods and services: food, energy, water supply, well-being and recreation, flood regulation, etc. However, this environment can be degraded by pollution or by developments (dams, dykes, navigation channels, sand and gravel extraction, etc.), leading to the alteration or even the loss of the functionalities and services mentioned above.

Worldwide, the WHO estimates that nine out of ten people breathe air containing high levels of pollutants. Similarly, 7 million people die each year from the effects of indoor and outdoor air pollution.

This contamination by pathogenic organisms can occur very quickly. A single intake of infected water can be enough to cause serious diseases[5] that are difficult to treat. Treating and monitoring affected populations using innovative and advanced technological means will therefore remain one of the main solutions.

4 https://www.aquaportail.com/definition-4437-ecosysteme-aquatique.html.

5 https://www.solidarites.org/fr/aider-plus-loin-temoigner/combattre-les-maladies-hydriques/maladies-liees-a-leau-lexique/.

1.2.3.2.2. Climate change

Climate change has the potential to increase exposure to disease transmission as a result of prolonged changes in the seasons.

The year 2020 has been classified as one of the three hottest years[6] ever recorded according to Météo France. During this same year, the UN warned that there was a risk that the mercury rise would exceed 1.5°C, a threshold set in stone in the Paris Agreement, by 2024.

This increase is likely to have both short- and long-term effects on the transmission of diseases spread by a specific vector. These include epidemics of infectious diseases, as well as certain animal diseases, in environments with high population flows. These epidemics are enough to convince us of the need to use innovative solutions to detect and trace infected people and to contain the spread of the resulting diseases.

1.2.3.2.3. Pollution and flooding

Floods regularly hit regions of the world, causing the spread of viruses and, by the same token, the spread of complex and transmissible diseases. Air pollution can have various short- and long-term effects on health. Air pollution in urban areas increases the risk of acute respiratory diseases (pneumonia, flu epidemics) and chronic diseases (e.g. lung cancer), as well as cardiovascular diseases.

Climate variations affect the prevalence of vector-borne diseases, such as yellow fever and malaria, and alter the burden of water-borne and diarrheal diseases, such as cholera and rotavirus infections.

Environmental crises such as pollution, heavy flooding and the ensuing illnesses of the affected populations are certainly pushing our decision-makers to think of innovative ideas to anticipate these types of crises. One such idea would be to encourage the high-level development of innovative initiatives driven by the evolution of information and communication technologies. We cannot talk about influenza epidemics without talking about the health crisis we are currently experiencing: the Covid-19 pandemic.

---

6 In the 120 years since national averages have been measured, nine of the ten warmest years have occurred in the 21st century and seven have occurred in the last decade.

2

The Covid-19 Pandemic, an Exogenous Factor of Innovation

2.1. Origin

The new coronavirus (SARS-CoV-2), which is at the origin of an emerging coronavirus disease (Covid-19), was first detected in the city of Wuhan, Hubei Province, China. It took a catastrophic turn with high incidence rates in China and subsequently spread across the globe.

2.2. How the pandemic began

At the time of writing, Covid-19 has caused the death of nearly 1.92 million people and the recorded infection of 90.3 million people. We would like to look back at some of the dates that marked the start of this pandemic, which in itself represents a real catalyst for a number of innovative health initiatives. The appearance of the first suspected cases of Covid-19 reportedly took place in Wuhan, China, in December 2019. Chinese doctors issued warnings about an unknown virus that had appeared in people working at the Huanan wholesale seafood market in Wuhan, Hubei province, in central China, where live wild animals are stored and sold. It turned out to be similar to the SARS epidemic that spread in 2002–2003 in China. However, it remains a mystery as to how and where the virus was transmitted to humans. A few months after the appearance of this virus in a

Chinese city, the coronavirus spread to other countries and across the world, resulting in a pandemic that has had serious implications for people's health and daily lives. Here are some historical dates on the management of the first wave of the epidemic in Europe.

2.2.1. *January 24, 2020: first cases of infection with the new virus in Europe reported by the WHO*

Two patients were detected in Paris and one in Bordeaux, according to the WHO, which added that all of these people had traveled to Wuhan, China, and were hospitalized in France. These different cases were diagnosed and quarantined. Subsequently, several cases were discovered in Italy a few weeks later. This is why the World Health Organization reiterated the need to put in place a plan to coordinate policies between States in order to define a roadmap to act effectively against this virus, stating that "the time has come to prepare ourselves"[1].

2.2.2. *January 28, 2020: implementation of the first measure of the European Union's health crisis management plan*

In the event of a health or environmental crisis due to a natural disaster (e.g. the tsunami that hit the Indian Ocean in 2004) or dramatic events (e.g. the attacks of September 11, 2001, the Madrid bombings of 2004), the European Union can implement several sectoral response procedures to facilitate the coordination of strategic decisions between States, the main goal of which is to remedy the situation.

In response to the Covid-19 outbreak, on January 28, 2020, the Croatian presidency of the European Union decided to implement an initial measure in this sense by activating the mechanism for political reaction in crisis situations (known as the integrated political crisis response (IPCR)) in "information sharing" mode. The role of this mechanism, which is integrated into the Council's crisis management plan, is to facilitate the coordination of health policies between EU Member States and affected Member States, EU institutions and other key players in the European Commission (EC). This tool exists in several modes:

---

1 Source: *Nouveau coronavirus : premiers cas signalés en Europe* (OMS) (un.org).

– tracking mode;

– information sharing mode;

– full activation mode, which prompts the EC to act in response to the crisis.

In response to the Covid-19 crisis, the EC opted for "full activation" mode on March 2, 2020 in light of the evolving pandemic.

2.2.3. *March 8, 2020: quarantine of the northern part of Italy*

To contain the spread of the pandemic, on March 8, 2020, the Italian government quarantined the Italian regions most affected by the coronavirus – namely, all of Lombardy, which is the economic capital of the country, Milan, the region of Venice, the north of Emilia-Romagna and the east of Piedmont – before extending this measure by decree the following day to the entire territory. Millions of Italians were strictly forbidden from entering and leaving these territories and were limited to staying within this area. The main objective of this draconian measure was to protect the health of the inhabitants of this part of Italy, their relatives, their parents and especially their grandparents. All schools, museums, sports halls, theaters and cultural centers were closed. All other public events, in particular cultural and religious events, but also private parties, were banned in the whole of northern Italy. Weddings and funerals were also suspended.

2.2.4. *March 10–12, 2020: financial support measures announced by the European Union*

The most affected countries of the European Commission called for coordinated responses at the European level. An initial meeting of the European Council took place on March 10 by videoconference, with the agenda of defining strategies to fight the pandemic. Three days later, the President of the European Commission[2] and the President of the European Council[3] made an initial statement focusing on the economic response to supporting the European States affected by the epidemic and their health

2 Ursula von der Leyen.

3 Charles Michel.

systems. In particular, it was decided to create an emergency fund of 7.5 billion euros, potentially increasing to 25 billion euros.

Other announcements were made concerning the banking sector – in particular, the postponement by 1 year of stress tests and on-site inspections, and the temporary easing of so-called Pillar 2 regulatory requirements. This easing was aimed at the euro currency zone and its impact is estimated at nearly 500 billion euros in reduced capital requirements[4].

2.2.5. *March 11, 2020: the WHO reclassifies the "epidemic" as a "pandemic"*

Initially called an "epidemic", the WHO now began referring to the situation caused by Covid-19 as a "pandemic". This status served to signal that the scope of the disease was broadening and thus to prompt accelerated policy decisions at the international level. "We have determined that Covid-19 can be characterized as a pandemic", WHO Director-General Tedros Adhanom Ghebreyesus said at a press conference in Geneva on Wednesday, March 11, 2020. WHO officials also called on the international community to strengthen its overall surveillance system to better protect hospitals, strengthen testing centers and put in place procedures to track contacts of infected people to stop the chain of transmission of Covid-19.

2.3. Covid-19: digital therapy as a response to the fight against the pandemic

In view of the brief history of the start of the health crisis due to Covid-19 that we have just presented, it is important to remember that it is a very contagious virus causing symptoms such as fever, dyspnea, asthenia, pneumonia and thrombocytopenia and that severely infected patients succumb to the disease. Coronaviruses were previously known to cause mild respiratory diseases in humans in some cases or severe infections in immunocompromised cases. Young people represented a demographic that did not display severe symptoms of the disease.

Nonetheless, the impact of the global Covid-19 pandemic has been marked by the rapid spread of the disease. The virus reached more than a

4 "Flash info : l'Union européenne face au Covid-19", March 2020, senat.fr.

dozen countries around the world in less than 6 months. Coronaviruses have the highest recombination frequency among all RNA viruses.

2.3.1. *Advanced imaging techniques for diagnosis*

Advanced imaging techniques, such as computed tomography (CT), magnetic resonance imaging (MRI), positron emission tomography (PET), single-photon emission computed tomography (SPECT) and ultrasound (US), are being developed to provide an answer to Covid-19.

Imaging has the advantage of being non-invasive and can detect signs of organ dysfunction at an early stage using clinical data. The results of qualitative radiology reports can be quantified using standardized techniques, including longitudinal image registration and organ lesion segmentation, which measure morphological and physiological changes due to disease. Artificial intelligence (AI) algorithms that learn from data can be unsupervised or supervised (e.g. in the case of deep learning), and the latter algorithms can be trained before being used on a database. Clearly, imaging data alone are not sufficient to train supervised neural network deep learning algorithms, as the imaging data must be labeled (e.g. pneumonia with normal X-rays, lesions versus normal tissue) to ensure the correct identification of the algorithm.

Molecular imaging is therefore a means to better understand cellular and molecular states compared to anatomical imaging, such as standard CT and MRI, which provide structural information for large volumes of clinical data.

According to the scientific literature, chest X-rays of affected patients show lesions in the lungs, with varying degrees of defects depending on the individual. In addition, each of the coronaviruses can cause severe lower respiratory tract infections. The disease affects all age groups and is exacerbated in people with underlying comorbid conditions.

To combat this virus, integrated advanced technologies are proving useful in detecting severe or asymptomatic cases.

2.3.2. *Telemedicine*

In terms of telemedicine, the Covid-19 pandemic has radically changed the way care is delivered in our health systems. To reduce the risk of transmitting the virus to patients or healthcare professionals during their practice, many visits have been postponed when possible and replaced with telemedicine consultations. Although many local and state restrictions on travel and non-essential services have subsequently been lifted, we can see that ambulatory practices have adapted to this new reality of remote medical care, developing new organizations and innovative approaches to delivering care.

2.3.3. *Smart epidemiological maps*

Many techniques based on artificial intelligence have been developed to interpret medical images and integrate intelligent algorithms of automatic learning associated with the convolutional neural network.

In addition, real-time epidemiological maps are being developed and made available to the general public. These maps automatically incorporate a proactive approach to case identification and the tracking of individuals, using remote monitoring devices for physiological parameters, such as temperature (including infrared scans, now required in all public spaces and transportation hubs), and travel history through connected objects and their mobile applications using single-cell sequencing. Importantly, human genome sequencing with structure predictions for the new coronavirus and its complex quaternary biomolecular structure can be successfully delineated in 2 h using machine learning algorithms.

2.3.4. *Detecting the virus using intelligent tests*

At the screening level, tests to identify Covid-19 positive cases are based on the reverse transcription polymerase chain reaction (RT-PCR) technique. Thus, the development of new approaches to detect patients with greater accuracy remains a major challenge.

2.3.5. *Treatment of the disease using simulation analysis and decision support techniques*

For the treatment of this disease, a technique based on artificial intelligence has been proposed. It can be used to analyze similarities and differences between treatment plans.

One of the difficulties faced by caregivers in treating patients is the limitation of equipment such as ventilation systems. Under such conditions, hospitals are faced with the difficult decision-making process involved in selecting which patient should be allowed to access such care. To this end, a multi-criteria decision analysis algorithm based on artificial intelligence has been proposed to hierarchize patients according to their health status.

At the diagnostic level, machine learning allows for the construction of a more accurate diagnostic model for Covid-19 patients based on observed symptoms and routine test results. Symptoms are in most cases gathered by asking basic questions of patients and by using data from emergency care admission tests.

2.4. Conclusion

It is expected that the Covid-19 pandemic will further accelerate "frontline" technological and logical innovations, and in particular the interest of industrial developers in creating innovative solutions, such as intelligent telemedicine platforms and e-healthcare monitoring applications, as all these innovations also help to reduce the costs of disease management. These applications often integrate intelligent algorithms.

These innovative solutions are leading to better coordination of care among healthcare professionals and the increased adoption of remote care, facilitating the shift to ambulatory care. It is also worth recalling that care in the patient's home can lead to better outcomes and greater efficiency. However, these new models will require continued attention from policymakers, investment from provider systems and rigorous scientific evaluation with the help of expert panels and learned societies.

3

Digital Therapy: For Which Health Needs?

3.1. Introduction

The components of a health system are the health needs of the population, its ecosystem of actors, its organizational strategy in terms of material, logistical and human resources, and its care methods.

The increasing health needs of populations are driving existing healthcare systems to innovate in their therapeutic and organizational strategies to deliver services that meet the stated expectations.

In order to innovate, it will not be sufficient to maintain the traditional approaches established decades ago. We could, for example, use the development of new information and communication technologies to propose innovative solutions that can optimize therapeutic approaches in order to guarantee effective and efficient care adapted to the current realities of our communities.

3.2. Background on digital health needs

Broadly speaking, the health needs of populations are closely related to the various crises mentioned in Chapter 2, including environmental, demographic and organizational crises.

These solutions are considered to have an added value that extends beyond the improvement of the care strategy under consideration.

Given the complexity typically associated with scientific medical management decisions in the management of certain health crises, competent governments face the dilemma of how to act quickly when their basic decision-making processes are based on deliberations balancing political considerations.

For example, some governments systematically adopt examples of policy decision-making models obtained from other countries.

In this respect, one of the objectives of this mapping is also to promote, through a detailed analysis, the major innovative national and international flagship initiatives in the field of health that clearly address a medical need within a population.

3.3. Expressing health needs within populations

In order to map innovative solutions based on artificial intelligence (AI) in the field of health, it is necessary to identify the different needs of populations.

These include needs related to improvements in:

– the organization of the patient's care pathway;

– the empowerment of the patient with respect to their own medical care;

– the valuation of the health professional's expertise;

– the quality of care provided by the healthcare professional;

– the opening up of intelligent support services for care centers;

– scientific research;

– scientific and technological monitoring.

Contribution level of the solution	Needs	Specialty	Design technology	Possible innovative solutions
Healthcare professional	Capacity building for pre-, peri- and post-operative care personnel in the treatment phase	Artificial intelligence (AI)	Automated data analysis	Microsensors for microsurgery support incorporating a machine learning approach
				Decision support platform for a therapeutic strategy integrating AI algorithms
Healthcare professional and patient	Remote consultations during the diagnostic phase	E-health	Telemedicine	Telemedicine platform assisted by passive sensors that transfer data
				Robotics-assisted telemedicine
				Telemedicine assisted by AI
Healthcare professional and patient	Strengthening of the follow-up of management		Remote monitoring	Mobile health applications through connected objects with geolocation
				AI-assisted patient monitoring platform
				Online remote monitoring platform
				Robotics-assisted remote monitoring platform
Healthcare professional, general public and patient	Improvement of medical knowledge		Training	Virtual platform for health acculturation integrating AI
				AI-enabled science advice management platform

<table>
<tr><th>Contribution level of the solution</th><th>Needs</th><th>Specialty</th><th>Design technology</th><th>Possible innovative solutions</th></tr>
<tr><td rowspan="2">Healthcare professional and patient</td><td rowspan="2">Organization of the shared digital patient record</td><td rowspan="2"></td><td rowspan="2">Digital patient record</td><td>AI-assisted online appointment scheduling</td></tr>
<tr><td>Robotics-assisted appointment scheduling</td></tr>
<tr><td rowspan="3">Healthcare professional and patient</td><td rowspan="3">Capacity building for pre-, peri- and post-operative care personnel in the treatment phase</td><td rowspan="9">Robotics</td><td rowspan="3">Surgery</td><td>Surgical robot</td></tr>
<tr><td>AI-powered assistance robot</td></tr>
<tr><td>Robotic limbs and exoskeletons</td></tr>
<tr><td>Healthcare professional and patient</td><td>Improvement of medical knowledge</td><td>Training</td><td>Robotics-assisted simulation platform</td></tr>
<tr><td rowspan="5">Hospital, public, patient</td><td rowspan="5">Strengthening of support services</td><td rowspan="5">Services</td><td>Reception robots</td></tr>
<tr><td>Automatic disinfection robot</td></tr>
<tr><td>Availability/recycling of medical equipment through robotic assistance</td></tr>
<tr><td>Drone for delivery assistance</td></tr>
<tr><td>4D printing</td></tr>
<tr><td>Healthcare professional and patient</td><td>Improved mental capacity of the patient for treatment, diagnosis or education</td><td>Virtual reality</td><td>Cognitive surgery</td><td>Immersive virtual reality platform</td></tr>
</table>

Table 3.1. *Identifying the needs of the population in terms of care*

3.4. Examining the proposed digital technologies

3.4.1. *AI-assisted remote patient monitoring*

In the era of the fourth industrial revolution, healthcare professionals increasingly need to have access to a significant amount of detailed patient data in order to optimize their medical care. At the same time, patients increasingly want to have access to more information about their pathology in order to be truly active and empowered when it comes to their healthcare. These patients may be, for example, elderly people with multiple co-morbidities (chronic obstructive pulmonary disease and renal failure, cognitive and psycho-behavioral pathologies, malnutrition, cardiac failure, diabetes) who require regular monitoring by healthcare staff.

Some health professionals are in favor of installing an intelligent circuit that would facilitate the remote monitoring of patients by continuously communicating large volumes of data on the physiological parameters of sick people.

This is how remote patient monitoring platforms are progressively appearing, the objectives of which are to improve morbidity and mortality, reduce hospitalizations and improve quality of life while reducing medical and economic costs.

This is a process that involves the transmission of data that constitute health indicators from the patient to the professional and the interpretation by a physician of the transmitted data.

3.4.2. *AI-assisted telemedicine*

Teleconsultations allow physicians to diagnose, treat or detect disease early. They thus facilitate the digitization of data for patients who might be at a higher risk of disease. On the other hand, diagnosis is a multidisciplinary process that includes a set of tests such as blood tests, imaging tests or neuropsychological tests.

In a telemedicine setting, innovative AI algorithms based on clinical data can provide a satisfactory solution incorporating machine learning. This type of modeling can produce more objective results while focusing on predicting disease occurrence for diagnostic purposes. Data-driven computational approaches can test combinations of data variables.

It should be noted that health data capture methods are critical to making the interpretation of data modeled on AI algorithms during a telemedicine consultation process more reliable.

3.4.3. *AI techniques*

With large volumes of clinical data, some AI algorithms can be useful in diagnosing and even predicting outcomes for many common conditions. To address the challenges of data reliability, availability and security, even more powerful and constantly evolving algorithms are being developed for data acquisition, processing, storage, display and analysis. We will come back to this in Chapter 4.

3.4.4. *Robotics technology in health*

The design of a new robot involves two major tasks, namely the mechanical design and the control strategy design. The first includes the production of a solution able to execute a set of actions. At this level, the designer should give a form of AI to this device so that it can perform the tasks that it has the potential to perform. For the design of control and monitoring strategies, prototypes are proposed that iteratively learn from previous versions until a certain prototype is acceptable and until this prototype becomes a candidate solution.

Setting up a scenario requires describing and parameterizing a scenario model for robotics simulation. Thus, the evaluation of candidate solutions in remote patient monitoring, robotic surgery or robotics-assisted telemedicine (in the automatic disinfection of infrastructures, for example) remains one of the challenges in the field of robotics. Robotics-assisted simulation is therefore highly appreciated for testing such solutions, as it enables the simultaneous verification of the quality of the output for remote communication, the tasks predefined by the designer, the assimilation of human language, etc. Robotic simulation also has the potential to thoroughly verify the existence of cybersecurity attacks by malicious actors. Simulation will also allow for the design of future intelligent robots that are even more efficient, especially since we will have benefited from the lessons learned during the simulation of previous versions.

The ability to perform scenarios that link robot and human highlights a new technology: self- or semi-autonomous remote surgical robotics. This will enable surgical operations to be carried out in collaboration with telepresence robots for patients with reduced mobility in less accessible areas. This technology may also prove to be very beneficial for medical teams who have patients to operate on remotely, like astronauts sent into space for advanced research purposes.

3.4.5. *Supply chain with drones*

The smart technologies identified will improve the management of the supply chain, specifically from the point of view of delivery and stock level monitoring. This delivery can be positioned:

– in an open circuit, that is, from the hospital or the distributor to the patient's home;

– in a closed circuit, from the distributor to the hospital, focused on support services, emergency cases, etc.

Drones are robots in the form of small unmanned aerial vehicles, generally controlled remotely by radio waves. They improve the management of the supply chain in the health field.

Their application can be very useful for the delivery of medical products such as blood samples, drugs, vaccines and human organs, especially in difficult-to-reach geographical areas.

Technically, the architecture of a drone includes the following elements:

– a plane without a pilot;

– a ground control station;

– a link to ensure the transfer of data (communication);

– the flight controller: this is the central data processing unit of the drone;

– the ground control station, which provides data to human operators. This is the information needed to control and/or monitor the unmanned aerial vehicle (UAVs) during their remote aerial flight;

– data links: these are wireless networks that ensure the control and transfer of the information flow between the drone and the control station.

Drones operate at different frequencies, and one of the challenges related to the use of this technology is anticipating the risks for the populations that are in the vicinity of a drone that has embarked on its flight path.

To this end, it is important to employ ethical and deontological guidelines on the use of drones in order to keep vulnerable people safe. These guidelines should be integrated into the design, production and marketing of these innovative devices. They should also take into account the risk–benefit ratio of their use, as it is always wise to weigh the opportunities and risks offered by a particular innovative solution. The advantages could be, for example, the reduction in delivery time, the delivery of a product in a context of shortage of regular delivery people, etc.

In terms of disadvantages, we can cite the risks to privacy and the confidentiality of patients' clinical data. In terms of confidentiality, there are three types of risks:

– the physical confidentiality regarding the capture of images and videos: a drone could be used to spy (by capturing images or videos without the consent of the nursing staff) on the work of a medical team in an isolated place;

– the confidentiality related to the geolocation of a patient: for instance, there is a risk that a patient who is heading to a private hospital could be monitored by a drone without their consent;

– the confidentiality of a patient's living environment: a drone can be used to monitor a patient's lifestyle from the air without their consent.

A further point about drone performance (the quality of service and silent flight) also remains to be put into context. Drones can also be used as vectors of a potential cyberattack (such as the installation of a faulty connectivity network to access the drone's data) by malicious users. There are also the risks of collisions between drones or any other device and/or flying animal.

It is therefore necessary to strengthen the techniques for effectively detecting drones, in health applications in particular. For example, we could develop robust techniques for detection by video, audio, radio frequency, radar, etc. In this sense, simulators are currently set up to identify wireless networks as well as drones in the vicinity. Since drones are now seen as a means of transporting healthcare products for first aid teams relieving traditional carriers, it is also important to set up a smooth traffic flow.

3.5. Mapping the population's digital health needs

There are numerous types of AI available to improve overall care delivery. Table 3.2 outlines the health needs of communities and how AI technologies are providing answers to address them.

Contribution level of the solution	Design technology	What changes with this technology compared to the existing one	Possible innovative solutions	Some success factors
Healthcare professional	Automated data analysis	Technology for the automatic detection and tagging of lung changes suspected to be caused by inflammatory, oncological or tuberculosis processes from a platform for analyzing CT scan data obtained by repeated exposure to X-rays. This platform incorporates artificial intelligence (AI) algorithms that help a radiologist easily recognize pathological changes in CT scans performed either on a scheduled basis or as part of mass preventive health screenings	Microsensors for microsurgery support incorporating a machine learning approach Decision support platform for a therapeutic strategy integrating AI algorithms	This technology, which incorporates AI algorithms, should enable healthcare professionals to make informed decisions and achieve optimal results more quickly, with a significant improvement in the rate of early detection of people with lung damage at the end of the chain
Healthcare professional and patient	Telemedicine	Telemedicine technology enabling the remote inspection of biosensor values, as well as text and video communication, with alarms on devices such as tablets and/or smartphones carried by hospital staff: – continuous measurement of physiological parameters; – message notifications on a mobile terminal; – video communication	Telemedicine platform assisted by passive sensors that transfer data	Reduction in the costs of care Solution to the problems related to medical deserts

Contribution level of the solution	Design technology	What changes with this technology compared to the existing one	Possible innovative solutions	Some success factors
Healthcare professional and patient	Telemedicine	Telepresence robots enable two-way communication and can be remotely controlled to provide support to isolated individuals by connecting patients with family members and physicians. Applied robotics is a leading technique in telemedicine today that has the potential to transform physical examinations and clinical care, as well as monitor patients in remote conditions. From a cloud platform, robots and devices in the patient's home can be managed. The robot can be programmed to help patients with mobility problems who wish to be assisted both in performing activities that keep them mentally and physically active and in keeping contact with their family or even receiving health services related to their diseases that monitor the evolution of these diseases and the patients' mental state and help them to perform specific activities in emergency situations	Robotic-assisted telemedicine	/
		Telemedicine technology that incorporates AI algorithms	Telemedicine assisted by artificial intelligence	

Contribution level of the solution	Design technology	What changes with this technology compared to the existing one	Possible innovative solutions	Some success factors
Healthcare professional and patient	Remote monitoring	This technology works from a personal portable electronic device connected to a mobile application. The application works in two directions: on the one hand it communicates data about a patient's body parameters for which specific alarm thresholds can be set; on the other hand, it can receive directions or instructions for the patient from the designated care provider. The mobile application is integrated with a web platform that is used both to collect data from the application and to send communications to the application	Mobile health applications through connected objects with geolocation	Includes connected medical devices in the care pathway Facilitates the remote monitoring of certain health parameters (body temperature, oxygen saturation via oximeter, heart rate, etc.) with the healthcare professional Addresses the challenges of the shift to ambulatory care Reduction of travel time through remote monitoring of physiological parameters Early detection (prevention) of certain diseases through data collected by the mobile health application Involvement of the entire ecosystem in the implementation of a new organization of care
		This technology enables patients to be monitored from home, alleviating the burden on hospitals. The technique consists of integrating advanced sensors and/or robots encompassing intelligence methods for the strict control of the patients' health condition in order to preventively treat a possible runaway disease. This allows for the timely delivery of effective medication. This technology also involves an AI-assisted monitoring unit that enables effective early detection capable of identifying the onset of criticality	AI-assisted patient monitoring platform Online monitoring platform Robotics-assisted remote monitoring platform	Mobilization of a team of health professionals (as well as a team dedicated to the maintenance of the solution in the case of failure) to remotely monitor notifications in order to react at the right time Given the evolution of a disease, this mode of surveillance will allow the medical community to manage the indiscriminate influx of patients in emergency rooms and hospitals

Contribution level of the solution	Design technology	What changes with this technology compared to the existing one	Possible innovative solutions	Some success factors
Healthcare professional, general public and patient	Training	A web portal for the training for healthcare personnel	Virtual platform for health acculturation integrating AI	/
		A web portal for publishing scientific audiovisual content with subtitles. The subtitling system uses artificial intelligence applications for automatic speech recognition (such technology will be able to support several languages). This platform allows the text to be edited and errors to be corrected. Once the edits are completed, the recording is automatically published	Platform for managing scientific advice with AI	/
Healthcare professional and patient	Digital patient record	Technology enabling appointments corresponding to the activity of the establishments to be scheduled online. This technology offers both online medical appointment scheduling editors and remote secretarial services in compliance with current regulations. Its essential functionalities are: filling in an online appointment form, managing cancellations, managing teams (patients and health professionals), data security and managing the rates linked to the office consultation	AI-assisted online appointment scheduling	The presentation of the human–machine interface (ergonomics: personalized presentation of health professionals' profiles, search engine, availability of customer reviews opinions, etc.), easy identification of time slots, health professionals' schedules, notifications on the availability of all appointment requests to be defined Need for regular updates and real-time management (absences, etc.)
			Robotics-assisted appointment scheduling	

Contribution level of the solution	Design technology	What changes with this technology compared to the existing one	Possible innovative solutions	Some success factors
Healthcare professional and patient	Surgery	Robotic technology providing greater precision and surgeon comfort and easier access to minimally invasive surgery	Surgical robot	Reduction in the number of "open surgeries" associated with greater morbidity Roll out of robotic technology to all surgical specialties
			AI-powered assistance robot	
		Robotic technology useful in the post-operation phase	Robotic limbs and exoskeletons	
Healthcare professional and patient	Training	New technology that provides the ability to create scenarios that link the robot and the human	Robotics-assisted simulation platform	
Hospital, public, patient	Services	Robotics technology allows for the design of reception/telepresence robots that can be used by hospital staff to visit patients while reducing the risk of hospital infections, especially for those who do not have access to the appropriate protective equipment. This technology is particularly based on the design of intelligent and fully open-source humanoid robots specialized in the interaction and manipulation of objects. These robots can also replace or assist healthcare professionals in specific tasks, considerably reducing the number of human interactions. During conversations with the patient, data are collected and analyzed from the cloud platform by healthcare professionals	Reception robot	In hospitals, we identified three factors: – patient monitoring so that any reduction in the frequency of patient visits would result in a decrease in the risk of exposure; – ceasing the use of personal protective equipment and hence the resolution of its shortage in many hospitals; – relieving hospital staff overwhelmed by the flow of patient files to be processed

Contribution level of the solution	Design technology	What changes with this technology compared to the existing one	Possible innovative solutions	Some success factors
Hospital center, public, patient	Services	Digital twin-based technology that includes a discrete event simulation model combined with an optimization algorithm that analyzes an image or surface from an electron microscope and estimates its ability to filter out hazardous atmospheres. In effect, this digital twin is able to simulate the disinfection process of an existing surface and run "what if" scenarios with different parameters to improve its effectiveness	Automatic disinfection robot	The process must be carried out in several places at different times Acceptability to caregivers Training of dedicated personnel
		Technology developed to provide visibility at a given point in time with regard to the availability of equipment. This can include the availability of beds not assigned to patients, with a forecast based on data analysis taking into account various parameters, including the stock status and an expiration risk assessment with an optimized suggestion on how to move or remobilize them. Risks related to the production and delivery of equipment and supplier viability through AI-based web monitoring can be identified by: – providing ongoing monitoring and reporting as the situation evolves; – sending alerts; – assessing potential impacts to allocate scarce resources to the most impactful areas and mitigating risks to operations to maintain production	Availability/recycling of medical equipment with robotic assistance	Optimal centralized visibility of the market situation of equipment and consumables used in healthcare centers, quarantine sites and warehouses Better follow-up of the traceability of the equipment (i.e. the equipment consumed, ready for use and remaining to be recycled)

Contribution level of the solution	Design technology	What changes with this technology compared to the existing one	Possible innovative solutions	Some success factors
Hospital center, public, patient	Services	This technology calls for the implementation of devices that can be remotely controlled or moved autonomously. They would have compartments for transporting biological samples with a secure opening system	Drone for delivery assistance	Establishment of management rules to ensure better handling of this technology by the personnel dedicated to its use. These management rules will be based on the following points: tests/reviews on the use of the drones, tests/reviews on the maintenance of the devices, training on how to use them, recurrent tests on the level of appropriation of the devices by the dedicated personnel Reduction of transport time of biological samples
		Digital platform with 4D printing to meet specific needs in the management of diseases. It is worth recalling that with 3D printing, objects are designed by adding successive layers of material. Four-dimensional printing adds the possibility of changing the color, shape or texture of a 3D printed over time depending on external conditions	4D printing	Improved management of serious clinical cases. Acceptability of the technology by healthcare teams Responds to needs from a virtual data hub Design plan for the solution adapted to the expressed needs Organization of tests/reviews of the prototypes
Healthcare professional and patient	Cognitive surgery	Platform integrating virtual reality methods and serious games applied to patients as well as health professionals. Such immersive technologies could improve collaboration capabilities both between patients and between physicians	Immersive virtual reality platform	Allows the professional to better understand the disease and to choose the most appropriate therapeutic strategy Supports the training of health professionals in certain specialties

Table 3.2. *Mapping of innovative solutions that integrate artificial intelligence algorithms*

3.6. Conclusion

It is worth recalling that, in some countries, diagnoses are often less adapted to the needs of patients. Due to the lack of appropriate tools, some healthcare institutions are slow to react to life-threatening emergencies, which often reduces the chances of survival.

Empowering patients through connected and intelligent medical devices is important. However, the volume of data collected for management becomes significant. It requires reorganization of the nursing staff to better follow the notifications issued by the patient as connected health objects that generate useful information for the monitoring of management are employed.

Most of the innovative technologies identified to meet the needs of the general public work with AI algorithms. At the same time, they raise a unique set of ethical, legal and policy issues that potential business models will need to address.

4

AI Techniques Involved in the Design of Innovative Solutions

According to the scientific literature, there is currently no precise and clear definition of artificial intelligence (AI), but we can note that it includes several areas whose general purpose is to analyze data while recalling that each field of AI gathers different methods with specific underlying theoretical approaches.

With high hopes and ambitious goals, AI has thus become an influential field with characteristics that can be used in the medical field. It is also likely to determine the evolutionary course of the healthcare system over the next 50 years.

The contributions of AI for the practicing anesthesiologist are considerable. The machine learning (ML) described above allows programs to learn and react to data without prior programming. The data that can be analyzed during the anesthesia process through ML is vast and includes, but is not limited to, digital data, images, text and speech or sound. Thus, for the anesthesiologist, AI can be used for anesthesia depth monitoring, anesthesia control, event and risk prediction, ultrasound guidance, pain management and operating room logistics.

In oncology, AI can be used to diagnose and classify cancers. In surgery, it can be used for the preoperative analysis of clinical data. In gastroenterology, AI can be used to detect a lesion in the gastrointestinal tract, while computer-aided diagnosis can interpret the image and provide an interpretation of the lesion.

We believe it is necessary to understand the useful AI techniques that can be used to significantly improve care.

As a reminder, a medical device by definition means any instrument, apparatus, machine, implant, in vitro reagent, software, material or other similar or related item. Such devices may be used by health professionals for the diagnosis, prevention, monitoring, treatment or relief of a disease.

In this chapter, a set of key AI techniques that support the design of smart medical devices are outlined.

4.1. Applied health techniques

AI can be defined as the study of algorithms that give machines the ability to model reasoning, make knowledge representations and perform cognitive tasks, such as problem solving, recognizing and learning human language and objects and decision making.

ICT developments related to Big Data and the ability to store, process and protect large volumes of data have been real catalysts for technologies supporting the ever-increasing popularity of AI in healthcare.

It is worth recalling that AI includes four sub-domains.

4.1.1. *Automatic learning*

ML is an essential foundation for designing AI-based algorithms in order to improve the quality of results. These algorithms can also meet ethical and regulatory requirements.

In healthcare, ML is used to diagnose, treat and predict disease by recognizing predictive patterns. Traditional computer programs are explicitly programmed with a desired target.

For example, an individual can generate a program to display:

– a good result, that is, a class label for answer (a);

– a bad result, that is, a class label for answer (b).

To predict or explain a particular phenomenon, ML can use either:

– supervised learning, which involves a training stage for the data network in which a tutor constantly indicates its errors in relation to the correct behavior. This approach corrects the errors during the learning process;

– a structure detected from a set of data; we speak in this case of unsupervised learning, where the learning process seeks to recognize the patterns automatically. This principle is most often used for the search for clusters (such as clusters of Covid-19 infections).

Supervised learning is useful for training an algorithm to predict an end result based on data (clinical data, a particular case in the health domain) whose interpretability depends on the evaluation of features. Unsupervised learning is useful to search for patterns in an existing database.

Another subfield of ML is reinforcement learning, which generates a program that performs a task.

It should be noted that these modern ML techniques, although they help to increase performance, do not allow for the possibility of explaining the resulting predictions.

4.1.2. *Natural language processing*

This is a subfield that focuses on improving the ability of an algorithmic program to understand human language in order to analyze large clinical databases at scale.

This field focuses on collecting unstructured data or information from shared medical records and scientific research journals. However, one of the limitations of this type of processing lies in the multiple variables of human language.

4.1.3. *Signal processing and computer vision*

Computer vision describes how a program is able to recognize and analyze images and videos.

These techniques are used in the performance of assisted surgical operations, remote patient monitoring, the search for candidate drugs, personalized treatments thanks to the collection of an increasing amount of data from Big Data, etc.

4.1.4. *Artificial neural networks*

To store, process and share data, AI systems use other algorithmic methods based on artificial neural networks, fuzzy expert systems (FESs), evolutionary computation and hybrid intelligent systems.

The set of techniques is shown in Table 4.1. Note that AI domains can make use of the hybridization of techniques approach.

This approach is based on the simulation of reasoning based on the available basic knowledge. Indeed, each subfield of AI has its strong points, but also significant limitations. The realization of hybrid systems is an approach that combines the strong points of each approach and obtains a symbiosis of even higher performances or at least a wider field of application of AI. Another very important aspect of the development of intelligent hybrid systems is their ability to acquire new knowledge from several different sources and to improve it.

In healthcare, several innovative solutions could be built on a hybrid approach involving AI processes, such as:

– hybrid ML systems combined with autonomous robotics to design solutions for predictive medicine;

– hybrid systems of natural language processing with signal processing for the design of assistance robots.

In section 4.2, we present several AI applications whose design requires a hybridization of several techniques.

Domains	Techniques/functionalities
Natural language processing	Syntactic analysis, lexicon, discourse
	Interaction, knowledge and natural language
	Speech recognition and machine translation
Human language	Advanced interaction, human language
Processing of signals	Speech, vision and object recognition and activities
	Recognition of activities
	Search in an image bank
	Search in a video bank
	3D reconstruction
	Spatiotemporal reconstruction
	Object tracking and motion analysis
	Locating objects
	Visual serving
Machine learning	Supervised/sequential learning: rules are defined from validated examples called learning databases
	Unsupervised learning: the model is free to evolve to any final state when presented with an item
	Reinforcement learning
	Transfer learning: the ability of a system to recognize knowledge from previous tasks and apply it to new tasks

Domains	Techniques/functionalities
Machine learning	Semi-supervised or partially supervised learning
	Process optimization
	Bayesian methods: probabilistic graphical modeling and data analysis
	Latent variables, topical models, causal models and time series
	Neural networks, conditional probability machine
	Predictor concepts: approach to adjust parameters and modify them progressively to minimize error
	Classifier concepts: to differentiate elements belonging to different categories
	Deep learning with the emergence of the availability of large massive databases (Big Data) and the acceleration of the computing speed of processors
	Data mining, methods of operations for decision making, diagnosis, simulation and control of a system
	Massive data analysis
Multi-agent systems (agent = software) or distributed artificial intelligence	Multi-agent coordination (multi-agent planning, multi-agent decisions)
	Distributed problem solving
	Architecture of modules that follow each other in a predefined order
	Multi-agent learning (language, platforms)
	Multi-agent simulation
Neurosciences, cognitive sciences	Understanding
	Simulation of the brain and nervous system
	Cognitive sciences

Table 4.1. *Summary of artificial intelligence techniques*

4.2. Examples of AI techniques in health

4.2.1. *Multi-agent systems for designing solutions for gene recognition through medical imaging*

These systems allow the construction of platforms for the collection of pseudonymized lung computed tomography[1] (CT) data, useful for disease detection and assessment and the prediction of appropriate responses to treatment. Specifically, a basic technical knowledge of AI, including ML and deep learning algorithms, and more specifically AI neural networks, can transform databases into analytical models that can predict serious diseases. Using ML techniques, clinical data are correlated with patient data. Deep learning then performs image description and can generate virtual CT images from MRI datasets. Natural language processing visualizes and interprets the clinical data using special software.

The impact of the treatment of certain diseases, such as the most serious cancers, on essential services is sometimes gigantic, and it is more necessary than ever to make informed decisions. The construction of a distributed AI simulator of the spread of cancer in the body could be very important. Such a technological solution would optimize the medical care of patients with very serious cancers.

4.2.2. *Multi-agent systems or distributed AI to enable the design of solutions for predictive medicine*

Since some diseases can only be controlled by thorough testing and immediate response, a hybridization of AI domains including multi-agent systems, or distributed AI, and ML, to which signal processing could be added, would allow the development of a web/cloud platform with services for the efficient execution of testing procedures and evaluation tools for competent authorities.

---

1 Also known as a "scan", computerized axial tomography or CT-scan, a radiological examination that captures detailed images of the human body in three dimensions.

4.2.3. *Autonomous robotics and signal processing for decision support solutions: diagnosis and therapy*

Based on these two techniques, at least two major problems facing hospitals and institutions in health crisis situations can be addressed. These include the lack of optimization of hospital first aid, especially when health professionals are overly exposed to potentially ill users with insufficient protection or resources. There is also the issue of the widespread quarantine of users, which also leads to the prolonged isolation of individuals from social interactions, which can have a negative impact on mental health.

The construction of a social humanoid robot that integrates robotic and signal processing techniques will help both as a receptionist in the hospital to clarify doubts and control the flow of new incoming users, as well as in monitoring and assisting the people most affected by a disease.

Hospitals typically face logistical problems beyond any crisis situation. Moving around a hospital to deliver medications, documents or blood samples takes a lot of time for every caregiver and nurse while also putting them at a high risk of infection by a pathogen capable of causing or breeding disease.

In this case, a solution capable of transporting different objects, such as medication, samples or food, into hospitals or similar environments could have a positive impact on patient management. This solution could be extended with functionalities such as thermal cameras or other health monitoring devices, helping caregivers and/or healthcare professionals on the front line.

The rapidly changing environment is pushing healthcare systems to automate, digitally transform and continuously adapt. Healthcare experts need a fast and agile way to create new and digital solutions. The lack of coding and automation expertise is pushing tasks onto IT experts, who lack specific knowledge of the sector and are not widely available.

Thus, a plug-and-play connectivity solution for robots (and other devices) would be able to seamlessly connect the hardware to the rapid application development platform. This solution could therefore be extended to automization and robotics solutions.

4.2.4. *ML and augmented reality for diagnosis assistance based on holomedicine concepts*

Only selected physicians conduct patient visits and admissions to protect other physicians from infection. These physicians may consult with their colleagues at any time, regardless of location, if they have questions or concerns in specific areas in order to maintain emergency care. If the physician/assistant has questions, they can call a colleague or a specialist through specially designed VSI Holomedicine glasses. The holograms, which appear as 3D objects in the colleague's space, are perceived through appropriate glasses like the Microsoft HoloLens. The colleague called obtains the exact field of view of the caller on their laptop or smartphone and can advise them optimally without being on site themselves.

4.2.5. *Natural language processing and ML for remote monitoring of physiological parameters*

In this case, we can cite, for example, the construction of a data/AI platform that allows data to be aggregated and then processed quickly.

4.2.6. *Robotics and human language for supply management*

Companion robots are particularly useful to fight against viruses without exposing humans, keeping them away from any possible contamination. This type of robot would be able to destroy pathogenic microorganisms present in the air thanks to an ultraviolet lamp (UV-C), which is integrated into it. Other robots would be able to assess distancing. For example, if the minimum distance is not respected, a warning could be emitted with a flash and an announcement issued to keep a distance of 2 m in order to avoid being infected with Covid-19.

4.3. Ecosystem of actors involved in the design of innovative solutions

Today, state policymakers are paying serious attention to the development and commercialization of solutions that improve healthcare. However, according to the World Health Organization, many existing health systems still manage health problems in a disconnected and fractured manner, and there is still a lack of coordination between providers, stakeholders, organizations and settings, as well as in the timing of care provided.

To this end, various actors are joining forces to co-construct digital technologies using AI algorithms.

These key players are mostly from the private sector (small and medium enterprises (SMEs), start-ups, etc.), the public sector and the academic research field. To this, we add patients and healthcare professionals who participate in the evolution of the solution. We recall that the notion of an ecosystem of actors in digital health technologies calls for several notions, notably those of interaction and collaboration between actors.

An industrial actor is considered as any structure, very small enterprise (VSE), SME, start-up or scale-up that represents a stakeholder in the construction of innovative solutions. We can mention companies such as:

– DARVIS Health in Germany;

– Methinks software in Spain;

– Shark Robotics in France;

– ContentWise BVBA in Belgium;

– Findest in the Netherlands;

– UiPath in Romania;

– SuccessData in the UK;

– Synergy Management Consulting Cyprus Ltd in Cyprus;

– Solteq Plc in Finland;

– Rulex Innovations Labs Srl in Italy;

– FLUIDDA NV in the United States of America;

– Block Gemini in the United Arab Emirates;

– Mirai Innovation Research Institute in Japan;

– Flow Robotics in Denmark;

– Logixlab in Malaysia;

– DMLAB in Hungary;

– Black Swan Lux in Luxembourg;

– HealthBeats in Singapore;

– Unacast in Norway.

This list is, of course, non-exhaustive; you will find all the players in the global mapping of innovative solutions that can help to solve major public health problems.

The European Union has initiated directives to facilitate cooperation between companies, universities, research institutes and medical institutions in order to improve the innovative capacity of digital health technologies.

These industrial promoters have invaded this market through company mergers and acquisitions. In order to maintain the competitiveness of their products, these players have invested in research and development strategies focused on breakthrough and incremental innovations. They have put in place significant innovative organizational approaches in order to offer solutions that have the capacity to meet demand.

Having opted for mergers and acquisitions strategies, these industrial promoters are now on a rapid growth curve. Those who have not made this choice find themselves overtaken by the competition.

As part of their marketing strategies, actors involved in the design and development of digital health technologies are implementing commercial policies that aim to improve their own brand image and establish productive marketing channels.

In terms of the maturity of this ecosystem of players in digital health technologies, it can be said that, given the intelligent medical devices validated by the competent authorities, most of the co-constructed technologies are not yet in the market launch phase. They are either in development or in the testing phase.

4.4. Some challenges of AI

As in all scientific fields, the implementation of self-learning in the medical field involves a number of risks, such as the risk of surveillance capitalism[2] and cyberattacks.

4.4.1. *Artificial form of surveillance capitalism*

Imagine if, when a patient with an infectious disease goes to a hospital for treatment, the doctor who treats them is able to accurately envisage how the virus is spreading in the body and the exact level of the patient's immune defenses against their illness.

Let us transfer this imaginary scenario to a framework in which, to ensure their care, the patient discovers a course of action in which they have continuous access to their health data in real time from their home, which they can then transmit to their doctor remotely. In this case, this course of action is the means by which surveillance capitalism can emerge, since health data must be collected to optimize diagnosis and anticipate a future serious illness.

In the case of ML/AI, there is a considerable challenge linked to an artificial form of surveillance capitalism that translates into an economic model that is essentially based on the collection of health data and the automation of care. This automation involves, for example, the design of intelligent platforms that record a certain amount of health data, which more often than not leads to the problems of mis-sold health data, the problem of confidentiality and protection against individual privacy and cyberattacks.

4.4.2. *Cyberattacks*

Cybersecurity is an approach that ensures the protection, confidentiality, integrity and availability of data in an information system. All the information systems of healthcare institutions in which intelligent connected medical devices are integrated are exposed to cyberattacks.

2 Surveillance capitalism is based on the instrumentalization of individual behavior.

The risks of a cyberattack are generally:

– phishing, that is, sending a fraudulent e-mail or SMS that seems realistic to the receiver because it uses stolen data;

– identity theft, where one feels that one is a victim.

Since zero risk is impossible, the approach taken by healthcare facilities that prescribe devices that integrate is to perform a comprehensive risk analysis of the infrastructure and networks made available to staff and patients.

At the end of February 2021, the French media revealed the publication on the Internet of a file containing the medical data of nearly 500,000 people. A publisher of software for healthcare institutions identified 28 medical analysis laboratories among its customers affected by this leak. The company has informed these laboratories.

4.4.3. *Cost of assessing AI-assisted technologies in health*

Digital technologies are generally protected by patents, regulatory approvals and investment requirements. Some breakthrough innovations that incorporate AI algorithms into their design are in demand to enhance surgical techniques. However, these require significant investment to bring them to market.

One of the factors involved in bringing an innovative device to market is its evaluation. This can focus on the quality, effectiveness, acceptability and cost-effectiveness of digital technologies. These aspects remain challenges to be overcome in order to enable the widespread adoption and diffusion of these emerging technologies. These digital innovations can change both the organization of care delivery and the preventive approach to disease. They are evaluated by gold standards and by competent health authorities. These evaluations generally involve clinical trials, which are necessary to assess the quality of a solution based on clinical data.

There are other approaches to evaluating digital health technologies. Examples include:

– Quantitative analysis (meta-analysis): this is a method that makes it possible to assemble the results of several studies to produce an objective synthesis according to a precise and reproducible protocol. It also makes it possible to quantify the overall result for all the studies considered. It responds to a precise method for the search, selection, presentation and analysis of available studies for a given question.

– Cohort studies: these studies can provide feedback on the use of digital technologies by patients.

– Databases and therefore clinical registries: these registries allow post-marketing surveillance and continuous evaluation of the efficacy and, most importantly, the outcomes of new treatments and technologies.

– Epidemiological studies: these studies aim to analyze the factors that influence the frequency or distribution of diseases and other health phenomena in populations exposed to these factors. They include experimental studies, non-experimental studies and prevalence studies.

– Studies based on medico-socioeconomic health issues: these studies make it possible to assess the advantages of emerging digital technologies over existing technologies, including their profitability in terms of economic and organizational gains.

All these approaches are costly and require investment from the industry.

5

Comparative Analysis of the Diffusion of Innovative Solutions between 2020 and 2030

5.1. Origin of the data for the analysis

The data for our analysis come from the OECD data platform.

This research was therefore carried out as part of an approach involving documentary research aimed at collecting data that shed light, in part, on the solutions put in place around the world to fight the Covid-19 pandemic. These solutions identified in our mapping constitute in themselves the basis of a new age of health, which is that of digital therapy.

The various initiatives were registered before June 1, 2020. For our analysis, we used the first 100 initiatives registered by industrial sponsors.

It should be noted that the data collected have limitations, as with any sample. The solutions that we observe and analyze may not have seen the light of day, as we do not have indicators that allow us to follow these projects from their launch to their completion, but it is possible that some of the recorded initiatives were launched over the course of 2020 and did not reach completion due to the lockdowns generated by the health crisis.

Based on our results, the best digital health solutions can be adopted in healthcare centers, in the pharmacy network and even in private homes. Change may be driven by a moral and compelling sense of the need for widespread implementation.

We can clearly expect a wider use of person-to-person health communication tools, effective tools like the remote infrared medical thermometer, various specialized sensors incorporating AI for rapid medical diagnosis and telemedicine terminals.

Medical teleconsultation services should be developed for the entire population in order to better support patients to manage their health and to alleviate the workload of physicians by providing personalized preventive advice.

There is also a need to implement solutions assisted by AI techniques to help senior citizens and people with disabilities living in isolated areas to master computer tools.

5.2. Data analysis

Figure 5.1 presents a diagram that shows us how technological solutions integrating artificial intelligence have evolved. We focused on a sample of 100 initiatives.

5.2.1. *View by country*

5.2.1.1. *Estimating trends in initiatives by country*

According to this chart, Germany comes in first among the countries in Europe, with 20% of digital health technology initiatives issued relying on AI applications. In second place is Spain, with 16% of its digital health projects including AI techniques. Belgium ranks third with 10% of its proposals. France is fourth with 7% of digital health projects relying on AI and the UK is fifth with 5% of digital health initiatives incorporating AI algorithms.

As the largest economic power of the European Union, Germany wants to position itself as a leader in the digitization of the care chain, hence its first place in this study. It is worth recalling that the digitization of the healthcare chain is one of the future projects of the European Union in which communication technologies, AI, robotics, data science and computer security are the driving technologies.

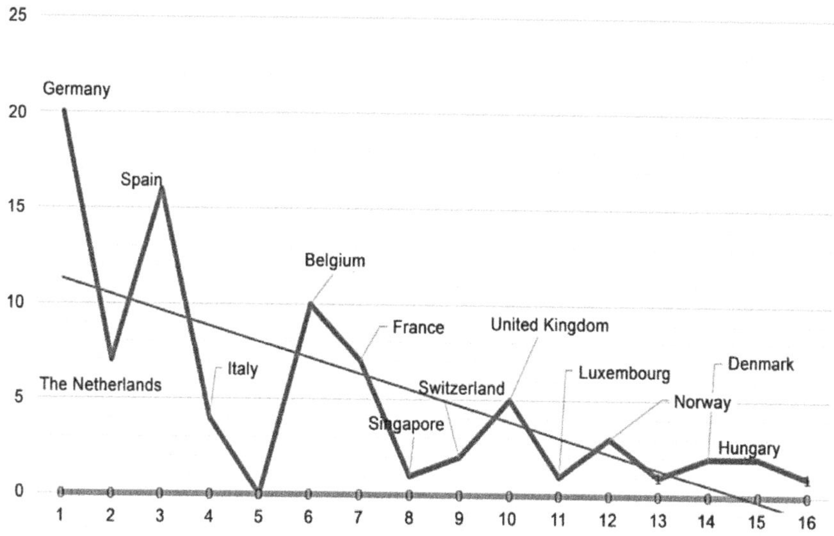

Figure 5.1. *Estimated curve of country initiatives in AI health. For a color version of this figure, see www.iste.co.uk/beyala/digitaltherapy.zip*

5.2.1.2. *Estimated trends in German AI health initiatives*

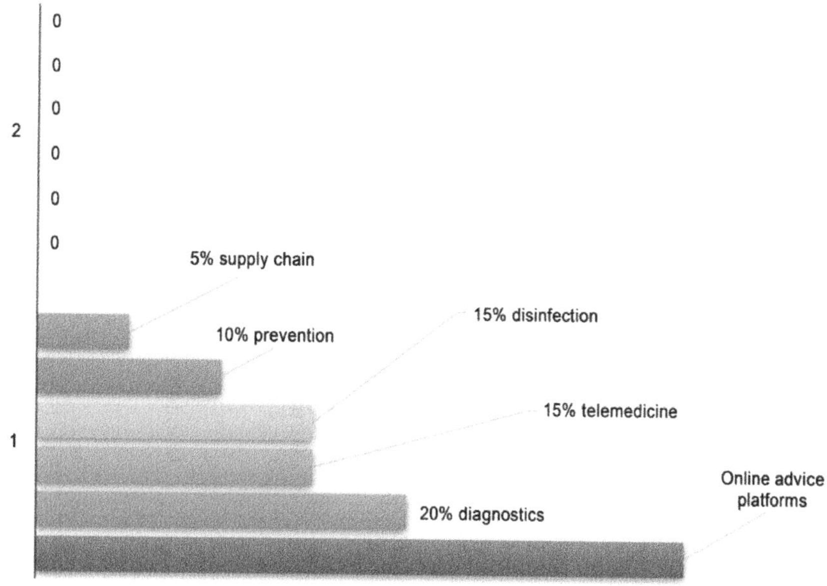

Figure 5.2. *Estimated curve of AI health initiatives in Germany. For a color version of this figure, see www.iste.co.uk/beyala/digitaltherapy.zip*

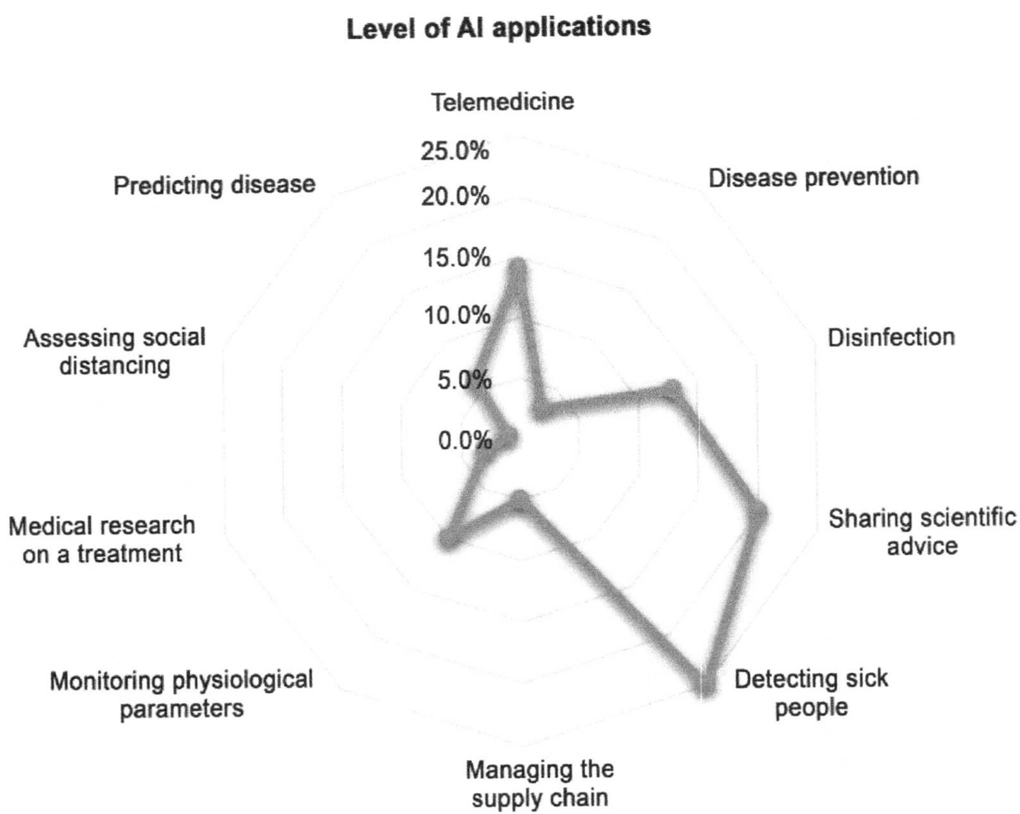

Figure 5.3. *Diagram representing the design levels of AI health applications*

From the diagram in Figure 5.2, it can be observed that German manufacturers are interested in designing a significant number of intelligent solutions to facilitate diagnosis, which accounts for 20% of initiatives. However, very few initiatives are registered in the construction of intelligent solutions to improve the supply chain of hospitals.

5.2.2. *General view*

In Figure 5.3, we present a summary diagram of the scale of implementation of AI techniques in health across the developed countries featured in our study.

5.3. Presentation of AI health initiatives

One of the objectives of our study is to provide a global vision of AI health initiatives across the world. In this section, we highlight the most highly developed AI health applications with respect to the health needs expressed by patients.

5.3.1. *Creation of platforms integrating AI*

Of the 100 innovative solutions proposed by the industry to solve major public health problems, 20% of future solutions involve the creation of platforms that would offer wide-ranging medical knowledge to EU populations, with qualified information from official sources consolidated in one place. This information could be customized by country or continent.

This figure is explained by the arrival of phenomena such as the cloud and Big Data. The adoption of these types of services allows our healthcare systems as well as the general public to store and follow scientific opinions produced by several actors. It is also important to mention that these platforms alone ensure the centralization, authentication, deletion and distribution of information in a digitized environment.

Cosibot is a platform developed by a German company that facilitates written and spoken interaction among people with visual and hearing impairments to enable them to access scientific information.

If all bodies of a healthcare facility were to face an increase in phone or email inquiries by several orders of magnitude, a conversational chatbot[1] informing users in several languages (English, French and Spanish) could provide reliable information to both requesting patients and official entities. It would be available 24/7 and accessible via websites, Facebook, WhatsApp and Telegram. These functionalities would be based on providing answers to citizens' frequently asked questions (FAQ) in real time in an automated way and thus avoiding false answers thanks to the truthful information supervised by a multidisciplinary team and led by experts in the health sector, the geolocation of users, data analysis and updated information on health measures. The virtual assistant would ingest millions of pages in real time with systematic updates for the virtual assistant based on data provided by the health authorities.

The mlx system proposed by a German company would allow scientific and distributed data sources to be collected and collated.

PIBNavi, which originated in Germany, also collects data from a variety of sources to predict key parameters of pandemics tailored to local circumstances, such as who to test first, measures that restrict the movement of people, etc.

Generally, all of these platforms would provide conversational AI capable of handling this task in real time, that is, 24/7. Moreover, they are designed to run very efficiently on a website or in a private cloud with no external application programming interface (API) required.

The AI techniques used are generally:

– deep learning, trained using a set of existing CT scans;

– predictor concepts;

– supervised learning;

– latent variables, topical models, causal models and time series;

– object tracking and motion analysis.

1 A chatbot is a software robot capable of conversing with a human in natural language. To chat, its user asks a question through a textual interface (SMS, instant messaging applications, mobile apps, etc.) or voice interface (connected speakers, voice assistants integrated into a mobile application, etc.).

Similarly, the most common application areas of AI in the creation of these platforms used to enrich our scientific knowledge would be:

– automatic learning;

– signal processing;

– multi-agent systems (agent = software) or distributed AI;

– robotics and natural language processing.

5.3.1.1. *Vulnerabilities of these solutions*

There are several possible risks when it comes to managing communication about scientific advice from smart platforms. These vulnerabilities could include identity theft, problems related to the spread of false information and any type of threat related to cyberattacks. Since this information is most often collected and stored in large databases, this could allow cybercriminals to hijack the data. There are also issues related to data confidentiality, as privacy concerns require a massive investment.

5.3.2. *Diagnostic assistance solutions using AI techniques*

According to the analysis of our mapping, 25% of the solutions integrating AI techniques would be diagnostic assistance solutions enabling healthcare professionals to analyze and detect a disease that would be harmful to a patient's health.

Cancer, for example, is the second leading cause of death worldwide, claiming 8.8 million lives in 2015 according to the World Health Organization. In 2017, only 26% of low-income countries reported having pathology services generally provided by the public sector. Less than 30% of low-income countries reported having treatment services, while the proportion for high-income countries exceeded 90%.

Ebola virus disease (formerly known as Ebola hemorrhagic fever) is a serious disease, often fatal in humans. The average case fatality rate is about 50%. In previous outbreaks, rates have ranged from 25% to 90%. The WHO strongly recommends the use of diagnostic tests that have had independent, international evaluation. The tests currently recommended by the WHO are either automated or semi-automated nucleic acid tests (NATs) for routine diagnostic management or rapid antigen detection tests for use in remote locations where NATs are not readily available.

In addition, according to the WHO, HIV remains a major public health problem of global concern, with 75.7 million (range 55.9–100 million) people having been infected with HIV since the end of 2019. The virus has caused 32.7 million (24.8–42.2 million) deaths since the end of 2019.

In view of the above figures, the players involved in the industrialization of digital health have been working together to develop innovative test kits that embed AI algorithms, and it is important to remember that the demand for intelligent diagnostic assistance solutions will increase in the coming years – even if we can already foresee a decrease in the rate of their productivity once the Covid-19 pandemic is over.

Driven by the need to facilitate medical care, diagnostic assistance solutions that integrate AI algorithms generally include cancer diagnostic tests, blood sugar monitoring tests, pregnancy tests, cardiology tests, hematology tests, infectious disease tests, sexually transmitted disease (STD) tests and sexually transmitted infection (STI) tests.

The Healthentia application allows individuals to report their health status by answering a simple evaluation questionnaire sent to their smartphone. This facilitates the monitoring of the evolution of the symptoms of a disease and allows for a diagnosis of the evolution of the detected disease.

Another medical solution could prevent false positives or false negatives in the results of certain medical tests, using an AI-based anomaly detection algorithm. Data would be collected on patients' symptom history and would help identify and predict results in new patients. The anomaly detection algorithm would suggest whether the test result could be wrong and whether the test should be repeated. The AI techniques used in this type of detection would be:

- supervised learning;
- some Bayesian methods;
- deep learning.

In Italy, the LEO console addresses the problem of operator safety when handling or moving infected material in hazardous environments. The LEO console, in fact, can be used to control any remote operation device, fixed or mobile, from a remote location. The LEO console is a lightweight, portable teleoperation console consisting of a stereoscopic vision system, two input devices and a foot switch. This console would provide a high definition stereoscopic view of the remote scene and two input devices. The AI technologies to design such a solution could be, for example, a hybridization of techniques including:

- deep learning;
- supervised learning;
- latent variables;
- topical models;
- causal models and time series;
- cognition for robotics and systems;
- design, perception, decision, action.

In Spain, to monitor and advise people who have been in close contact with a person infected with a contagious disease, as validated by a doctor, one company is proposing to improve the process of testing scans. The results are stored in a database integrated with an application. All data are encrypted and stored on a local database that would only be used in the event of an infection to analyze the data and inform those who may be infected. It would be an app on Android and iOS where you would have to register using your phone number.

The purpose of the application is to be able to recognize and connect to other devices, regardless of the platform, and exchange information with a view to facilitating the research on contact cases.

In Germany, to monitor the main vital parameters of humans (pulse, respiratory rate and temperature), special equipment is usually required. One proposed solution would be to have an integrated monitoring system capable of identifying the vital parameters of several people in a room at the same time. In addition, people's movements as well as their location in a room could be detected, while protecting their privacy, and the data could be consulted locally or remotely.

Such a technology would be designed based on the following actions:

– deep learning;

– supervised learning;

– latent variables, topical models;

– causal models;

– time series.

The functionality of this application would ensure the unparalleled interpretability, explicability, traceability and reproducibility of the data originally implemented, which could help users to make better data-driven decisions and automate a number of essential tasks in medical care.

In Japan, a solution has been implemented that consists of an autonomous robot that can be placed in a designated area (e.g. a shopping mall) and monitor a people's body temperature, identify people with a fever, approach them and launch a teleconference with a doctor. It works using an autonomous navigation system to patrol the designated area, AI to detect people and a thermographic camera to monitor people's body temperature, interacting with anyone it deems to have a fever. Based on machine learning, the AI techniques used would be:

– an understanding of human language;

– deep learning, which would be trained on a set of existing CT scans;

– predictor concepts;

– supervised learning;

– latent variables, topical models, causal models and time series;

– an object tracking algorithm and motion analysis.

Despite the strong growth of intelligent diagnostic solutions, it is important to remember that the current regulations governing the development and marketing of these solutions remain very cumbersome. This includes the lengthy approval process for these solutions by the relevant authorities, which could hinder the progress of this emerging sector.

5.3.3. *Creating intelligent solutions for medical research*

Note that 3% of the solutions integrating AI techniques are solutions that would allow medical research to progress.

In France, My Data Models uses the latest advances in AI, specifically machine learning, to build interpretable models of data. By reviewing these models, researchers can find patterns and discover new correlations. The solution is used daily in healthcare to diagnose cancers and propose drugs to patients with rare diseases.

5.3.3.1. *Creation of telemedicine solutions embedding AI techniques*

Note that 14% of the solutions integrating AI techniques are solutions that would allow telemedicine procedures to be performed.

This figure can be understood in terms of the increase in the use of e-health applications by hospitals, clinics, research centers and patients. The impact of the coronavirus crisis is a considerable asset for the growth of this field of e-health. Primarily due to the lockdown measures imposed by most states, the monitoring of patients from their homes has increased significantly as a very significant proportion of the population is reported to have widely adopted telemedicine procedures. In addition, there have been recent changes in the regulations in force that favor the digitalization of medical care. They put into practice favorable predispositions on the reimbursement of telemedicine acts by accredited organizations. This change of context has made the population more aware of certain advantages of digital health. As a result, this should generate considerable investments in this field of medicine, not to mention the involvement of an even greater number of players in order to promote the research and development of intelligent technological solutions that can be easily adapted by end-users.

In France, Ubbo, a telepresence robot, facilitates mobile online video communication between remote people. With its rotating and tilting head, it ensures a bi-directional audio/video communication while protecting caregivers. It is also envisaged to be used for pre-diagnosis by patients themselves or with the help of a nurse using the Medvir diagnostic application. This would reduce the time spent by patients in emergency departments and regulate incoming patients.

The solution has been developed from intelligent robotics. The techniques used by its industrial promoter would be:

– cognition for robotics and systems;

– design, perception, decision, action;

– interaction with the robots.

In Spain, the social humanoid robot PAL Robotics ARI helps, on the one hand, as a receptionist in the hospital to clarify general queries and control the flow of new incoming patients and, on the other hand, with the monitoring and assistance of patients with serious illnesses who need to be put into isolation.

This solution addresses at least two main issues facing hospitals and institutions:

– the lack of optimization of hospital first aid, especially when healthcare professionals are overly exposed to potentially ill users with insufficient protection or resources;

– the widespread quarantine of patients also results in the prolonged isolation of individuals from social interactions, which can have a negative impact on their mental health.

This ARI social robot therefore has the potential to provide telemedicine procedures and offer continuous social interactions. This robot can be updated with these additional features.

Among the technical means used for its design and development, we can mention:

– cognition technology for robotics and systems;

– design, perception, decision, action;

– interaction with robots;

– Bayesian methods;

– supervised learning;

– recognition of activities;

– speech recognition;

– machine translation.

As pointed out in our book *Connected Objects in Health: Risks, Uses and Perspectives* (Beyala 2017), one of the most critical risks for the user relates to the confidentiality of the data generated by a connected medical device. The solutions we have just listed embed AI algorithms and present serious risks related to the breach of individuals' personal data.

5.4. Overview of health AI legislation

As innovation in AI-based technologies is freely advancing in both healthcare and society at large, calls have grown for regulatory oversight to monitor, support and direct AI-based innovations and their application in society.

5.4.1. *European approach to AI regulation*

Comparing the current regulatory landscape for AI technologies to the "Wild West", the European Commission launched a white paper on AI[2] in February 2020 to outline a strategy for regulation and investment in AI technology to bridge the gap between regulation and this technological innovation.

The document seeks to establish a "high-quality" regulatory framework to orchestrate the "AI ecosystem" for the benefit of the healthcare sector and industry at large. The EC follows a generally ethics-focused line in its regulatory proposals in which risk assessment and the consumer protection imperative take precedence, stipulating the human oversight of systems and security requirements for large datasets.

5.4.2. *Regulating and supporting AI in healthcare*

The EC has made healthcare one of the main beneficiaries of the new regulations. The health sector can, in the words of the EC, "benefit from the data revolution" through more efficient and accurate diagnosis at a lower cost, among a host of other benefits.

---

2 Available at: https://ec.europa.eu/info/sites/info/files/commission-white-paper-artificial-intelligence-feb2020_en.pdf.

By placing healthcare at the heart of the AI ecosystem, the EC plans to strengthen the current use of AI across the supply chain, in AI-driven medical research where the development of additional tests and experiments will be prioritized and in the expanded use of robots in the provision of professional services in healthcare delivery.

AI technology is increasingly being used in radiology departments, for example, to diagnose patients more accurately by comparing screening slides with large datasets of previously diagnosed cancers. These datasets and the application of AI technology will be subject to new regulations to be implemented in the coming years.

5.4.3. *Scaling up AI regulatory policy in line with medical practice*

Instigating clear liability rules will be imperative as the use of AI increases in healthcare. Medical liability will need to be clearly defined as clinical decision making becomes increasingly automated.

The requirements for human oversight will go some way to ensuring that liability remains clear-cut, although the growth in medical negligence legislation reflects the difficulties that exist in determining liability.

Thus, significant work remains for the EC in drafting a set of regulations that address the controversy of existing issues regarding medical risks and technological applications. Moreover, as advances in AI technologies and their application continue to rise exponentially, the legislative task may exceed the capabilities of the European Parliament's new special committee on AI[3] .

5.4.4. *Reception of the regulatory proposals*

Stakeholder responses to the consultation for this white paper published in February 2020 were nevertheless largely supportive of the regulatory proposals. Of the 1,215 respondents representing academics, industry groups and citizens, support for the various GDPR-style regulations on

3 Available at: https://www.europarl.europa.eu/news/en/press-room/20200615IPR81228/parliament-sets-up-special-committees-and-a-permanent-subcommittee.

accountability and security ranged from 83% to 91% depending on the requirement. There is a clear appetite for change. Only 3% of respondents indicated that the current legislation is "fully sufficient", and an overwhelming majority called for a new regulatory framework or significant changes to the current legislation.

Although overwhelmingly supported by stakeholder groups, the EC nevertheless faces a considerable regulatory task in the disparate and divergent development and application of AI. Even when it focuses solely on the health sector, a comprehensive regulatory framework will require extensive ancillary legislation to ensure that policy responds to a constantly evolving practice, and new modes of regulation, as suggested by Ghebreab (2021), may be necessary.

5.5. Conclusion

As the Covid-19 pandemic continues to disrupt healthcare delivery in most countries around the world, e-health, telemedicine and even robotics applications continue to take center stage to support remote patient care. All these techniques are expected to revolutionize the medical world. The scientific advances presented throughout this chapter will probably have a considerable impact on the field of medical research.

Some technology solutions incorporating AI-driven algorithms will enable comprehensive screening for emergency care. AI is driving a suite of detection tools that will allow healthcare professionals to perform therapeutic analysis remotely, allowing patients to avoid physical contact with their doctor.

To this end, a huge advance in clinical research is expected thanks to AI algorithms. Microprocessors can simulate cells and organs of the human system so that drugs can be tested with very little risk to human or animal subjects, making clinical trials more efficient and accurate.

On the other hand, intelligent real-time diagnostic devices will cover considerable needs for a successful care pathway and will reduce the complexity of medical procedures and analysis.

Artificial intelligence also offers medical robots, which are necessary for patients to perform a pre-diagnosis by themselves or with the help of a nurse using a specific diagnostic application. This will undoubtedly reduce the time spent by patients in emergency departments and regulate incoming patients.

As governments restructure healthcare to meet the needs of populations, the above solutions may be critical to enabling a permanent transition to remote monitoring and screening, reducing the burden on waiting rooms and improving access to healthcare.

Regulatory barriers are likely to be an issue. For example, in the United States, regulatory discord among states has hindered telehealth adoption through prohibitive reimbursement and licensing regulations.

Yet telehealth represents a key opportunity to provide healthcare to people who have difficulty accessing health centers, and this is even more critical as we think about the new post-Covid reality.

In view of the above, we can conclude that even if science does not have the capacity to be a political tool, it can nevertheless guide political action in order to put in place the measures it deems necessary. These choices are difficult, because they place life, death and economics on the same level while taking into account that the resources allocated to healthcare systems are limited and that these systems can become overwhelmed.

PART 2

Digital Therapy and its Transformative Approach

6

Strategies for the Sustainable Adoption of Digital Health Innovation

6.1. Introduction: adopting digital health technology

The healthcare system is a set of services that is constantly faced with the challenges of efficiency, equity and quality, given the changing needs of the population. Thus, health systems in most countries require constant innovation to control costs across the range of services, improve knowledge in the scientific research environment and develop more effective and efficient mechanisms to improve the quality of care.

In the service of health, digital technologies have the capacity to improve access to care by providing an answer in one way or another to the problems of an aging population and the high prevalence of diseases. They translate into the use of intelligent assistance robots, intelligent surgical robots, robotics-assisted remote monitoring platforms, telemedicine platforms integrating passive sensors, mobile health applications connectable to connected health objects, artificial intelligence for the interpretation or automatic analysis of clinical data and so on.

It is worth recalling that there are different theories that can be implemented to enable the adoption of digital health technologies, namely planned behavior theory (PBT), diffusion of innovation theory (DIT), the theory of reasoned action (TRA), the technology acceptance model (TAM) and innovation adoption theory (IAT). Among them, the TAM is the most influential model for the adoption of a specific technology.

It is to this end that a number of developed countries have begun to embrace digital health to provide better quality health services to their patients.

Healthcare personnel, patients, their families and the general public are increasingly recognized as stakeholders who can play an important role in improving healthcare services. This may include the design and development of innovative solutions to problems related to usage. However, little is known about the role played by patients or the mechanisms by which they can help to facilitate the adoption of digital technologies in a complex healthcare system. As a first step, it would be desirable to identify the flows of expectations of all the actors involved in the digital therapeutics ecosystem.

In this chapter, we highlight the drivers of digital health adoption both by patients as well as by hospitals in developed countries.

6.2. State of the art of digital health advice

6.2.1. *Digital technologies for more efficient quality of care*

The population in most developed countries is aging. Digital health technologies play an important role in addressing the high costs of managing certain chronic diseases. Industrial developers are becoming more mature in their design of passive sensors integrated into smart devices to ensure the better monitoring of care. From these sensors, health professionals are able to make much more differentiated diagnoses compared to usual practices, which consequently leads to considerable savings in terms of costs via early diagnoses of chronic and complex diseases, for example.

Digital health technologies allow for the improved coordination and consumption of health service offerings based on the use of connected health software or applications.

6.2.2. *Hospital at home*

With the spread of innovative solutions, the delivery of health services could be transformed in the long term. We will move from the hospital outside the home to the hospital at home. This new form of care will minimize the interaction between the caregiver and the patient. Mobile health, or digital health, opens up a new dimension for healthcare systems that will change the existing medical offerings.

With the delivery of medicines to the patient's home, the industrialization of healthcare will remain an interesting sector for pharmacies in the long term. Today, the activities of pharmacies are still focused solely on the sale of medicines and certain medical devices. However, the arrival of connected health objects is shaking up the codes of the health market, giving pharmacists the opportunity to sell connected medical devices for remote monitoring. Pharmacists are therefore gradually replacing the family doctor and are arguably predestined to sell medical devices to the general public. They could therefore, in the very near future, make therapeutic recommendations in the care pathways of their patients.

6.2.3. *Evidence of sound and reliable comprehensive scientific data from the use of digital health technology*

It would be of great interest to have a repository of reliability criteria for the quality of data generated from digital health devices. Health professionals are generally busy with health consultations and taking care of their patients. They are not always able to inform themselves about digital tools of proven scientific quality. Since digital health technology (DHT) powers the collection of health data through data platforms stored in the cloud, it needs scientific evidence to be disseminated, adopted and even paid for. Thus, it makes sense to clearly prove the benefits of DHT. This will likely lead to the mass adoption of this technology.

This adoption will strongly depend on the level of maturity of data protection rules.

6.2.4. *Societal beliefs*

DHTs generate different opinions from the public. As a reminder, it is important to make the point that while DHTs can help doctors to make their diagnosis, they are not intended to replace them. Even if the digitization of the care chain has great potential through the integration of artificial intelligence techniques, as far as the analysis and interpretation of health data and medical decision making are concerned, doctors will remain in their place and will be the ones to make the final diagnosis.

It can be seen that older people are more often than not less experienced in the use of DHTs, which in the long run will lead to a two-tier society.

Take, for example, the wireless vital signs monitoring system. It is an integrated web-based software system that consists of several components, namely remote physiological monitoring devices (biosensors) worn by patients, a web-based graphical user interface used by both the physician and the patient himself/herself, a database server and a back-end web server. The system uses the hospital's wireless network infrastructure. It monitors health indicators including body temperature, blood pressure, pulse, temperature, electrocardiogram, oxygen saturation and respiratory rate. It is a DHT that allows for the monitoring of a patient remotely, continuously and in real time. It is generally beneficial for providing services regardless of the time or the location of the patient. It is a cloud-based platform materialized through a public website. Patients with urgent medical needs have to create an account on the platform's website before scheduling a consultation. It should be noted that these patients may include elderly people. During the registration process, each individual has to fill out a short form providing basic demographic information. A secure link is sent to the individual's email address to activate their account. Once the account is activated, the individual indicates to whom the electronic visit is directed and the type of provider intended (e.g. family physician). The website provides information about medical specialties not supported by its platform. Once the individual verifies that they are aware of their personal health information, they are asked to complete a series of short forms about the reason for the appointment, medical history, pharmacy selection, provider selection, payment and confirmation.

Technically, each patient carries an RFID tag for identification. In the traditional approach to patient monitoring, patient health data are tracked manually by the caregiver and in some cases by the patient. With this remote monitoring system, digital graphs of physiological parameters are generated automatically, replacing patient records managed manually by nurses. The system also allows healthcare professionals to view these digital graphs in real time.

This process of creating an account and logging in to the site may be difficult for older people to do. The adoption of such an innovative solution may therefore depend on both the patient's living environment and their geographical location. Hopefully, social polarization will push patients of all ages to become familiar with the same level of quality in terms of medical follow-up, especially when it comes to remote care.

6.3. Theory of adoption of health technology solutions

Even if it is noted that the health crisis caused by Covid-19 has accelerated the adoption of digital tools in the medical care of patients, it is agreed that the theory of adoption of technological solutions for even more efficient medical services is based on the following factors:

– the introduction of financial variables that would allow the costs of the services brought by the new technologies to be compared with the existing costs;

– the development of policy theories that would increase the creation of innovative solutions and facilitate their diffusion;

– the different characteristics of the ecosystem of actors;

– competition on the market in connection with the industrialization of the medical sphere.

In terms of strategic theories, we are thinking in particular of the unified theory on the acceptance and use of technology.

This theory was developed by V. Venkatesh, D. Davis and M. Morris[1] to explain the intentions of the individual end-user in the use of an innovation and their resulting behavior.

The WHO reminds us that the healthcare system is the set of institutions, people and resources involved in the delivery of healthcare. To talk about the healthcare system is to ask about a value chain that is in constant flux, with services moving and changing in space and time.

1 Venkatesh, V., "UTAUT, TAM 3, Modèles unifiés d'acceptation des technologies", *SI et Management* (sietmanagement.fr).

It is essential to keep in mind this dynamic approach of a care system in order to better calculate the dimensions of the collateral effects of technological leaps[2].

These different elements will undoubtedly be of interest on several levels:

– in terms of the attitudes of the patients who are the end-users of these innovative solutions;

– in terms of the barriers to adoption of these solutions.

6.4. General factors in the adoption of DHTs

In the medical field, technology is evolving in several ways. For example, it can evolve in terms of its uses and their acceptability by the medical profession, as well as by patients and their families. It can also evolve in terms of the technical performance of the tools it produces. At the level of existing systems, the organization of care is finding it increasingly difficult to respond to the rapid development of digital solutions.

One reason is that not all players in the DHT ecosystem have the same level of understanding of the benefits of NST. Most need time to understand the wide range of opportunities in emerging technologies. They need to develop their knowledge by seeking professional support.

The adoption of DHTs can be promoted by implementing the following points:

– reliable health data generated from innovative solutions;

– a communication strategy adapted to each country by influential groups and the media for all the opportunities related to DHTs that would enable support for patients, providers and even the government that finances certain care services;

– patient lobbying to better represent patient needs and expectations;

– strong governance to establish long-term perspectives for the use of digital health technologies;

2 A technological leap is, in a technical field, a major innovation in the design of a product. It corresponds to a revolution in the state of the art in this field.

– training of the actors involved to overcome the obstacles that could arise from the use and adoption of these DHTs;

– innovative approaches among stakeholders to break down rigid structures and enable them to easily integrate digital health solutions within their organizations;

– new approaches to cooperation between providers, patients and insurers.

6.5. Ecosystem of actors promoting the adoption of technology initiatives

When we speak of a system of care, we are referring to an ecosystem of actors, stakeholders and relationships that, when in action, provide care to patients, create economic value for participants, serve the interests of government and meet the needs of society.

6.5.1. *Ecosystem of actors for the adoption of a health innovation*

6.5.1.1. *Health professionals and patients*

A health professional is a person who exercises skill and judgment and provides a service related to the maintenance and improvement of the health of individuals or the treatment of injured, sick, disabled or infirm individuals by providing care and therapy.

Health professionals include physicians, nurses or any actor trained to participate in the medical management of a patient.

6.5.1.2. *Governmental authorities*

The role of government authorities in the adoption of innovative technologies is significant on several fronts, including as policymakers and as payers of public expenditure for population health. Most of the investment in health system infrastructure, including health workers and facilities, remains with the government.

Government authorities are also involved in the design of modern health systems by adapting them to new changes brought about by disruptive innovations.

6.5.2. *Adoption of digital technology by patients and the general public*

Many theoretical studies seek to describe the dynamic process of adopting innovations in the medical field. However, little is known about the factors related to decisions to adopt innovations and how the probability of adopting innovations can be increased.

It is believed that the involvement of patients in their care and their ability to play an important role in improving the learning of their physicians would lead to a scientific paradigm shift in which the patient's voice would be at the heart of an emerging era of participatory medicine. This would generate a positive impact, to which the engagement and involvement of patients in healthcare would make a significant contribution, whether in the understanding of their health condition, the way they can be treated and managed or through self-management and peer learning.

Patients are increasingly taking it upon themselves to set research agendas, including by suggesting research questions, serving on research teams and evaluating results.

6.5.2.1. *Adoption of digital technology in the hospital*

A number of technology determinants have been shown to influence the organizational adoption of new technologies, including their perceived usefulness, perceived ease of use, system compatibility, system security and IT infrastructure. New technologies are more likely to be adopted when an organization believes they offer more benefits than existing systems.

Healthcare institutions are gradually adopting new digital health technologies in their patient management processes.

Physicians are very important stakeholders in the development, adoption, use and choice of disruptive innovations. As coordinators and providers of patient care, healthcare professionals want to use innovative solutions in their daily activities, which would have a positive impact on the spread of these solutions.

They are healthcare professionals who use innovative solutions and most of the time have a scientific orientation in their practice. They are aware of the quality of the health data that a technology could generate as well as the efficiency that can be generated by the use of these emerging solutions. The roll-out of a digital technology by a health professional could also be due to their desire to increase their knowledge in the use of a new technology that would bring about considerable added value in the care strategy put in place.

Thus, physician acceptance is a key condition to ensure that the expected benefits will be realized.

At the same time, limitations in the adoption of digital technology in hospitals are thought to be related to the following factors:

– A lack of competition between city hospitals and private players: in many countries where service provision is privatized, private sector companies are forced to innovate in the traditional market or face the erosion of their position in the global market. This approach, which is essentially based on the desire to innovate when faced with the competition, is not yet visible in the health sector in most countries.

– The challenges of cooperating in a new virtuous ecosystem: in developed countries with complex and traditional healthcare systems, cooperation between healthcare institutions, public institutions, learned societies and industrial actors is often difficult because of the complexity of these organizations and the number of stakeholders.

– Resistance to the paradigm shift by some health actors: a change in society's behavior and a change in the habits of stakeholders will also be necessary to spread the positive effects of digitization of the healthcare chain, even though some countries are not yet sufficiently equipped to embrace the change brought about by DHT. In this context, the industrialization and digitization of healthcare is often met with a strong culture of resistance to change on the part of stakeholders.

– Stakeholders' expectations in terms of medical solutions are constantly evolving: while some countries maintain an international reputation for their quality of care, the needs of their populations are changing. Solutions to these expressed needs may entail significant costs for their development and deployment. In this case, the idea of "doing more with less" offers a tremendous opportunity to increase the financial sustainability of healthcare systems in some countries and enable the rapid adoption of DHTs.

6.6. Conclusion

Well-executed coordination and health data exchange are essential to internalize the added value of new digitally supported healthcare environments and ecosystems. The introduction of the Swiss electronic patient record will be an important step forward, but it only provides a formal framework for an advanced playing field of healthcare actors. The adoption of different types of digital health solutions does not necessarily disrupt the healthcare system but transforms it to some extent. Governance at the different levels of the health system plays a central role in balancing the different interests of stakeholders and the multifaceted impacts that emerge from changing conditions. Digital solutions promise to increase efficiency, contribute to treatment effectiveness and improve the way patients and healthcare providers communicate. However, these solutions will not necessarily solve the system burden caused by emerging societal needs and changing disease prevalence.

7

Indicators of Change in Healthcare Systems

7.1. Introduction

The first step is to identify the main determinants of the medium- and long-term evolution of the healthcare system, which will in turn lead to the evolution of digital health. Among the many factors that can be identified today, five have already been identified here, including:

– economic and political changes;

– the internationalization of economic activity.

7.2. New governance that calls for the consolidation of a hospital business model

Independently of the health needs implied by the demographic indicators mentioned above, the digital health system is also being transformed because of economic factors (profitability of Medtech or e-health companies, for example) and political factors. Digital health and its services (augmented humans, repaired humans, e-health, artificial organisms, connected patients, etc.) are directly concerned by these changes because of their important position in the socioeconomic and political scene.

It is estimated that the French e-health market was worth just over 4 billion euros in 2020. Beyond the context of Covid-19, 100 million euros have been set aside to accelerate the digital transformation of healthcare institutions, as well as 50 million euros for the deployment of telemedicine to finance the necessary digital equipment: consultations, payments and the remote reading of health insurance cards. In this respect, the ageing of the population, the challenge of distributing public spending, the need to harmonize the supply of care and the security of health data are all factors that require care methods and processes to be adapted.

The economy of the e-health sector, for example, is experiencing exponential growth due to the digital transition and innovations in clinical research to manage and support patients with chronic or infectious diseases. Bearing in mind that the computerization of the management and digitization of records began in the 1970s with the development of new information and communication technologies, we have now reached the creation of the shared medical record (*dossier medical partagé* (DMP)), which is already used by more than 6 million patients.

If we go back to the field of e-health, there are now more than 15 billion connected objects in the world, more than triple the number almost 10 years ago, and about 200,000 health applications. Their growth is exponential and some estimated their number to be between 50 and 80 billion in 2020, which means that each person in the world would own an average of six connected objects.

Moreover, the collection of data that is mass-produced nowadays makes it possible to compile not only the medical and behavioral information of patients, but also genetic information. The combination of Big Data and powerful computational algorithms would allow the creation of medical profiles and possibly the establishment of predictive patterns to anticipate certain pathologies.

In addition, there are strong barriers to entry in e-health when it comes to bringing a concept to market. For example, it is necessary to have a marketing authorization, or a classification when it is a medical device, one or more data security features that comply with the GDPR and clinical studies carried out in a hospital environment to prove the effectiveness of the device.

All of these requirements mean that start-ups wishing to enter the sector have to invest significant amounts of money upstream of the product development phase, often even before generating any revenue. However, in other sectors, the question of investment comes later; e-health/Medtech start-ups are therefore forced to find partners/investors early in their lifecycle and sometimes to rethink their operations and business model.

In order to implement these requirements, start-ups generally call on investors (business angels, specialized organizations, etc.). The latter can impose structural and financial constraints, notably on the nature of their business model and on their profitability (time, threshold). In addition, since the user does not usually pay directly, it is the intermediary organizations that finance the products or services. These are healthcare centers (public and private), health insurance organizations or complementary healthcare associations. The business model of start-ups and scale-ups must therefore be adapted to each organization and to their different structures.

As e-health start-ups face significant barriers to entry, in the coming decade the main socioeconomic evolution of digital health will concern the consolidation of a business model for hospitals, which is the biggest challenge for their development. Moving toward a model based on a fixed fee and the quality of care administered could be a solution envisaged by the State to support both healthcare establishments in their digital transformation and start-ups in their development in the field of healthcare, particularly in hospitals.

7.2.1. *Case study: Canada*

At the biotech level (in response to Covid-19[1]), the introduction of new regulations in Canada to reduce the price of patented drugs could "weaken" Canada's research-based pharmaceutical sector, the industry warns. Under the amended regulations, the Patented Medicine Prices Review Board (PMPRB) will have to decide whether the price of a drug reflects its true value and the ability of Canadians to pay by:

– considering the pharmacoeconomic value of each drug (based on its efficacy), the size of the market in which it is sold, Canadian GDP and GDP per capita;

– changing the list of countries on which it bases its price comparisons by removing the highest cost countries, Switzerland and the United States, and adding six lower cost countries (Australia, Belgium, Japan, the Netherlands,

---

1 Source: https://ici.radio-canada.ca/nouvelle/1705879/industrie-pharmaceutique-prix-baisse-reglement-delai-pandemie.

Norway and Spain). According to Ottawa, the new list will better align Canadian prices with the average prices of the OECD;

– requiring patentees to provide information regarding discounts and rebates to their customers in Canada.

The announced changes are scheduled to come into effect on July 1, 2020. The changes to the rules governing the prices of patented medicines are intended to lower those prices for the benefit of Canadians. The PMPRB protects and informs Canadians by ensuring that prices of patented medicines sold in Canada are not excessive and by reporting on pharmaceutical trends. Canadian prices for patented drugs are among the highest in the world. They are the third highest in the OECD.

7.3. Internationalization of digital health activities

In light of the current health crisis, the internationalization of activities related to digital health is more than ever at the heart of everyone's daily lives and will remain a key factor in the future economic recovery (particularly because this will mean an increase in imports of goods and services in this field of health) and in the sustainability and growth of start-ups, SMEs and large groups. However, profound changes are foreseen. The cards will be reshuffled and redistributed. This is an opportunity for those who will be the first to understand the new rules of the game and to adapt their international practices accordingly; it will be a disaster for those who are slow to integrate them.

7.3.1. *Case study: France*

The French government has put in place a support plan for companies advocating the industrialization and digitization of export healthcare to enable them to retain their customers, stay on top of their markets and remain competitive in order to seize the opportunities of the upcoming rebound. These emergency measures are essential and will certainly have to be adapted and supplemented as the situation evolves and as companies encounter difficulties and opportunities.

It is therefore necessary to anticipate changes, to consider new approaches to exporting and internationalization, and to adapt support tools in order to offer French companies the analyses and solutions that will enable them to face this crisis in the long term and to bounce back even more strongly internationally.

This is a change that has already begun in the organization of the economy and will accelerate in the coming years. For several years, some multinationals investing in digital health have been trying to reduce the dependency of their production lines on the Chinese economy, with the aim of regaining control in the most strategic sectors. Covid-19, for example, will probably accelerate the phenomenon of "nearshoring"[2] (the gradual return of part of the final assembly capacity to areas closer to the major consumer basins).

7.4. Conclusion

By digital health services, we mean a set of services composed mainly of online health services (allowing users to carry out one or more procedures in a dematerialized manner) and digital tools (connected health objects) for coordinating care and exchanging or sharing information, mainly intended for health professionals.

Ensuring state control of the digitized health system remains a dynamic and classic approach implemented in developed countries. One of its objectives is to rationally organize the response to the health needs of the population through technological innovations in health in the event of a threat. This is gradually being put in place in most countries of the world and presupposes a social system that values the development of new information and communication technologies in the community. This valorization requires the adoption, acceptance and diffusion of new technological solutions capable of providing better services in terms of medical care.

In particular, this policy is in favor of imposing a regulatory framework for the various uses and representations of these innovations on individuals within the framework of a rationalization of innovation.

2 Nearshoring, as opposed to offshoring, is the relocation of an economic activity to another region of the same country or to a nearby country.

State control of digital health services is exercised in several ways:

– either directly, with the State as the exclusive operator of digital health services (as in the United Kingdom);

– or indirectly, through the close control of parastatal (or even private) structures to which the services are entrusted under management (as in Italy).

A professional body of administrators specifically trained to work in digital health is responsible for managing, financing and planning the services expected by the population to meet specific needs, such as those exposed during the Covid-19 health crisis. The close proximity of these oversight bodies to political power puts strong and sometimes rapidly changing constraints on the system.

8

A Radical Change in the Care System

8.1. Introduction

Despite the presence of some flaws in our healthcare systems, there is an ongoing evangelization of the medical world evidenced by an increase in patient empowerment, a desire to move from disease-centered care to patient-goal-centered care and a growing interest in minimally disruptive medicine.

By the mid-2020s, the situation of our healthcare systems may have changed abruptly. In this scenario, practitioners would be more and more sensitive to the impacts linked to the adoption of new technologies, while patients would acquire a maturity in the use of innovative solutions and would become more active and involved at the forefront of their care.

Against the backdrop of today's healthcare system, we have the tremendous dedication of healthcare personnel who fight to save lives on a daily basis, as medical practices, research and solidarity undergo changes and restructuring. Public organizations, private companies and volunteers are coming up with an increasing number of creative and sometimes effective initiatives to respond to the immediate needs of patients by relying on innovative technologies such as e-health and telemedicine. Thus, it is possible to foresee the evolution of digital health, taking into account its contributions in effectively meeting the needs of patients.

The purpose of this section is to explore the drivers of the transformation of our healthcare systems by identifying plausible consequences.

The strategic interest of this reflection is to choose the approaches that determine the new age of digitizing health systems. These approaches serve primarily to reinforce the adaptive capacity of an organization in the face of future changes: they simulate these changes and their consequences by allowing institutions to simulate their recommendations and to develop their policy strategies in relation to the medical domain.

8.2. New organization of the health system

Despite the scourges of SARS, MERS and Ebola, to name just a few of the more recent pandemics and viral disease outbreaks, we have seen that we need to work together with health authorities and governments around the world to rethink our priorities for investing in healthcare systems. Among the changes that need to be made is the plan to create a single cloud to accelerate medical research.

8.2.1. *Creation of a single European cloud for medical care and research*

On March 13, 2018, a workshop was held at the EU Commission's Directorate for Health and Directorate General for Research and Innovation to assess the feasibility and challenges of establishing a health research and innovation cloud that would be accessible to researchers and health professionals across Europe, in line with the recommendations for a Euro-Mediterranean Innovation Council and the Horizon Europe 2021–2027 framework program.

In order to anticipate and prepare the medical community for future epidemics, it would be wise to encourage all scientific researchers to share data and best practices transparently across the world through a single data sharing platform. This would be a very important line of development for a system revolution.

The creation of a unique European cloud, extraterritorial and structured on open scientific data, which would bring together the knowledge and know-how of health professionals, would be a real asset; technological innovation in medicine will follow a pattern and a rhythm that will not only depend on the need and demand for healthcare, but also on the knowledge available in real time.

Access to a single, secure and equitable data platform for scientific information and research results during crises (Ebola, Covid-19, etc.) for researchers, media, medical staff, the general public, patients, etc., would be of the utmost importance to obtain accurate and affordable scientific answers. This would include clinical, epidemiological and laboratory data. Investing in a stronger and more resilient intercontinental health cloud system, capable of rapid and integrated responses based on the latest scientific findings, with equal access across the EU, is of crucial importance.

According to a new report from Science Business[1], as well as an independent group of cloud experts from academia, industry and the public (sector institutions), this project represents one of the strong policy priorities to be addressed by the new European Open Science Cloud Executive Board.

It is also clear that significant scientific progress is most often dependent on the volume of data and knowledge exchanged across international borders. At the same time, the Executive Council should consider how to achieve reciprocity and ensure that all parties accessing EOSC services comply with European laws on the protection of sensitive health data. The group also urges the new Board to prioritize the development of a sustainable business model and a strong legal and governance structure.

In the very recent past, most of the world's healthcare systems were characterized by a trend that led to a reduction in hospitalizations per capita, on the one hand, and to the strengthening of large healthcare centers, on the other hand. This process of concentration, which brings more quality, competence and advanced technologies, could therefore be accompanied, in principle, by an increase in the value of primary care in order to provide comprehensive care as close as possible to the citizen. However, in reality, in the case of complex care processes (Ebola and Covid-19 are examples), a significant gap remains between the communication of scientific research via dedicated sharing platforms and coordination in care settings.

In the context of the health crisis caused by Covid-19, factual data platforms have been set up to identify and analyze behaviors and representations of the impact of the crisis on the population. For example, one has been designed by the Human Science Research Council (HSRC) in

1 A unique forum that brings together leading organizations from industry, research, innovation and policy making at both European and national levels.

South Africa. To this end, an online survey was conducted to better understand people's behaviors and current patterns. As of March 27, 2020, approximately 2,400 people had completed the survey. The sample size was increased, and a statistician was assigned to assess the quality of the responses and data required to conduct the analysis.

8.2.2. *Creation of a "one-stop shop" per continent for the development of research and development programs*

Research and innovation (R&I) plays a key role in addressing chronic disease epidemics and virus outbreaks (e.g. Covid-19), particularly in providing science-based solutions, including an improved scientific understanding of diseases and the development of targeted treatments and diagnostics.

In addition to the multiple standard instruments of current and future R&D programs, we believe that it would make sense to set up a "one-stop shop" per continent co-financed by a multilateral initiative (see, for example, the Global Fund that invests in the fight against AIDS, tuberculosis and malaria, diabetes and cancer) with an open list of topics, among which a place should be reserved for the development of technologies aimed at supporting the preparedness and resilience of health systems and at increasing social cohesion through intelligent and person-centered primary healthcare.

This one-stop shop for R&D programs for each continent could also be implemented through more targeted investments in specific studies through, for instance, financial, administrative and voluntary initiatives, not only for the public sector but also for science-intensive companies.

One of the main recommendations for the proper functioning of this one-stop shop for research by continent would be to set up digital systems for the online evaluation of research proposals and their peer review.

In the coming years, we can expect a further increase in the digitization of science and the economy as a whole, as well as a strengthening of the role of governments in scientific affairs. This may involve a revision of priorities for the development of new health technologies.

These research programs will contribute to an increase in the development of autonomous production technologies both in the context of the reindustrialization of healthcare and for robotization in the healthcare services sector.

8.2.3. *Changing rules in the calls for projects*

Given the current demand for care, introducing changes in funding rules and/or conditions and procedures to speed up processes and streamline administrative procedures for calls for proposals would be an advantage. It would be imperative to streamline the launch of European, regional and national research calls or proposals in order to significantly reduce the grant period. Intensifying transnational cooperation as a way of sharing knowledge and information on needs and capacities would contribute to more effective protection of patients seeking innovative and adapted care.

Similarly, the relationships between caregivers, hospitals and health data hosts determine several characteristics of the healthcare system. For example, in France, a decree governing the organizational and operational measures of the healthcare system required to deal with epidemics in the context of a state of health emergency was published on April 21, 2020. This text specifies which data can be accessed, under certain conditions, by the State's "Health Data Platform" and the *Caisse nationale de l'assurance maladie* (CNAM). The French Data Protection Agency (*Commission Nationale Informatique et Libertés*, CNIL), which has given its opinion on this text, will subsequently carry out a more detailed analysis of this platform in the context of the uses envisaged that are not related to health crisis management.

8.2.4. *A new strategy for the production of scientific content*

In order to provide real information and undermine false beliefs about science, health authorities may undertake a cross-sectoral public science communication and public awareness strategy. This strategy includes specific elements:

– First, the production of digital infographics and videographics based on technical contributions provided by high-level experts from different States participating in a series of dialogues. This information would be the result of an analysis of data collected by different actors, presented in a way that the public would find educational and easy to understand. This type of material would be published in collaboration with various actors in the systems of care and other government entities via websites, social networks and other digital media in order to empower the populations that access and share this content.

– Second, the creation of live participatory dialogues with experts. These spaces would allow experts to resolve some of the most common misunderstandings with examples and technical explanations. For this exercise, users could submit questions via social networks, promoting a participatory and dynamic dialogue where citizens are represented.

– Finally, special editions of a dozen different texts and associated audio-visual materials would provide an opportunity for in-depth reading about a particular health situation through the perspectives of different related fields of knowledge. This material could, for example, be published in collaboration with stakeholders in the state healthcare system ecosystem and other government entities, including the Department of Health, and shared via their digital media to broaden its public reach.

8.2.5. *A new strategy to accelerate digital health innovations*

One of the major impacts of the health crisis has been the massive use of digital health by French healthcare professionals and patients. The growth of these uses has been made possible by, among other things, the lifting of certain legislative and regulatory barriers in the context of the state of health emergency, such as for telemedicine.

As we know, technological innovation in medicine follows a pattern and a rhythm that depend on health needs, but also on the dynamics of medical and technological knowledge, as well as on the industrial and commercial opportunities that may arise. These innovations, even if they do not meet an immediate need, are likely to create a demand for services among the population: in this sense, technological innovation contributes to shaping the health system, including its value system.

For some areas of digital health, the adaptation of the new legal framework is still insufficient to allow patients and/or healthcare professionals to fully develop therapeutic strategies adapted to their needs.

Thus, at the end of this health crisis, a return to the past for digital health uses is not an option. On the contrary, the coming months must allow us to take stock of digital health practices by analyzing and designing more solutions that allow the medical profession to operate in a new and more efficient way, as well as measures that have not been implemented but whose value has been fully demonstrated during the lockdown period.

8.3. Conclusion

Using the information available today, our analysis shows us that all the health, social, economic and ideological movements of tomorrow are already identifiable today. At the end of this book, we can foresee the beginning of a new age for the eco-digitized healthcare system predefined in the 1980s that would include all the recommendations learned from the different pandemics while still bringing radically different solutions to meet the needs of populations.

Appendix

Mapping Digital Innovations in Health

Here, we present a summary table of upcoming digital innovations in healthcare between 2020 and 2030.

For a color version of the table, see www.istecouk/beyala/digitaltherapyzip.

Identification			Expression of need		Application of AI		Performance and purpose	
Industry/ company	Country	Expectation of the solution	Expression of the identified need	Proposed solution	Field and/or means of application of AI	Possible techniques and/or actions	Alerts and/or features	Service rendered in the therapeutic follow-up of the disease
Reinhold Technik GMBH & Co KG	Germany	Robotic control of a virus	Covid-19 infections in bakeries and supermarkets at the point of sale/checkout	Development of a camera system that attaches to the ceiling and continuously checks the minimum distance from shoppers to the point of sale/cashier	Robotics	Design, recognition, action and decision	If the minimum distance is not respected, the buyer is warned with a flash and an announcement to keep a distance of 2 meters in order to avoid being infected with Covid-19	Disease prevention
divVoice	Germany	Voice command in service robots	Preventing exposed persons from having contact with surfaces	Voice and remote control of equipment in hospitals	Human language	Speech recognition and machine translation	Disinfection and sterilization to limit the spread of viruses	Disinfection

Identification			Expression of need		Application of AI		Performance and purpose	
Industry/ company	**Country**	**Expectation of the solution**	**Expression of the identified need**	**Proposed solution**	**Field and/or means of application of AI**	**Possible techniques and/or actions**	**Alerts and/or features**	**Service rendered in the therapeutic follow-up of the disease**
PICC SOLUTION	Switzerland	Management of scientific publications	Collecting scientific publications via a platform	PICC AI. Provision of medical knowledge to the professionals who need it with automatic translation of documents into 26 languages	Distributed intelligence or multi-agent systems	Platform languages	Selective sorting of documentation from a platform	Communication of scientific advice
Organon Analytics	India	Tracking the spread of an AI-based virus using telecommunication signals	Tracking the contagiousness of the virus by identifying where and who the virus can spread to using AI and the cell phone signals of infected individuals	Collection of cell phone numbers of Covid-19-positive test subjects from phone base station signals. The data sources are processed with artificial intelligence algorithms	Signal processing	Object tracking and motion analysis. Temporal and uncertain reasoning. Constraint programming	Cell phone users are notified of their likelihood of exposure. Locations/points with the highest risk of exposure are highlighted. These notifications would be the basis for proactive testing or prioritizing resources	Disease prevention

Identification			Expression of need		Application of AI		Performance and purpose	
Industry/ company	Country	Expectation of the solution	Expression of the identified need	Proposed solution	Field and/or means of application of AI	Possible techniques and/or actions	Alerts and/or features	Service rendered in the therapeutic follow-up of the disease
Lucentia Lab	Spain	Platform for Big Data and artificial intelligence	1) Self-diagnosis mobile app using the geolocation of individuals 2) Chatbots to address key concerns 3) Blockchain to certify patient veracity	The collected data would be processed to make them usable by artificial intelligence engines	Machine learning. Signal processing	Syntactic analysis, image and video bank search	The appropriate set of algorithms would be selected for training and to predict subsequent outbreaks and the main care needs by area	Monitoring of physiological parameters
Organon Analytics	India	Detection of anomalies regarding the Covid-19 test results	To avoid false positives or false negatives in the results of certain medical tests, an AI-based anomaly detection algorithm could be used	Data on patients' symptoms in the past would help identify and predict outcomes in new results. The anomaly detection algorithm would suggest that the test result could be wrong and that the test should be repeated	Machine learning	Supervised learning. Bayesian methods. Deep learning	Helps detect false-negative patients and prevent the spread of the virus in these cases	Detection of sick people

Identification			Expression of need		Application of AI		Performance and purpose	
Industry/ company	Country	Expectation of the solution	Expression of the identified need	Proposed solution	Field and/or means of application of AI	Possible techniques and/or actions	Alerts and/or features	Service rendered in the therapeutic follow-up of the disease
Pragmasoft Sp. zoo	Poland	Measurement of temperature	Automatic detection of human body temperature abnormality. Detection of infected persons with symptoms of a high temperature	AI models used for human detection, face tracking, body temperature estimation. This solution consists of thermal imaging sensors and AI models capable of measuring the human body and informing the individual in the case of a detected anomaly	Signal processing and machine learning	Searching in an image bank. Searching in a video database. Supervised learning. Classifier concepts. Transfer learning	A diffusion of sensors is ensured. An alert is signaled in cases of high temperature with notifications such as email, SMS and push notifications	Detection of sick people
contextflow GmbH	Austria	Medical imaging	Lung CT image patterns and GGO distributions are useful in the diagnosis of Covid-19 infections; contextflow SEARCH and TRIAGE have the functionality to detect them	contextflow platform for the collection of anonymized Covid-19 lung CT data. Useful for training and evaluating detection algorithms with its proof of concept partners and its extensive hospital network	Multi-agent systems or distributed artificial intelligence. Signal processing. Machine learning	Searching in an image bank. Searching in a video bank. Object tracking and motion analysis. Classifier concepts. Deep learning and data mining	Based on a sorting function for image patterns and on disease patterns, allowing infected people to be detected	Detection of sick people through medical imaging

Identification			Expression of need		Application of AI		Performance and purpose	
Industry/ company	Country	Expectation of the solution	Expression of the identified need	Proposed solution	Field and/or means of application of AI	Possible techniques and/or actions	Alerts and/ or features	Service rendered in the therapeutic follow-up of the disease
SAI BV	Netherlands	Physical activities	Keeping citizens healthy and physically and mentally active while in quarantine	ABLE is a voice- and text-activated AI tool that was created to match user needs with physical and mental training data. It alleviates isolation and loneliness during periods of quarantine	Human language and/or neuroscience, cognitive science and signal processing	Advanced interaction. Comprehension. Activity recognition. Searching in a bank of videos and images	Creation of a database of habits that would give advice (info on the spread of the virus) and establish relationships. Sharing of specific content (video, images, podcasts, etc)	Monitoring of physiological parameters
Alias Robotics SL	Spain	Cybersecurity using robot immune system	Most robots, including those most used in healthcare operations, are not designed with safety in mind, and this is often a top priority for vendors, according to a study by Alias Robotics	Managing adverse events related to robotic care from an application that captures myriad PCs in the NHS	Robotics and machine learning	Cognition for robotics and systems. Predictor concepts. Transfer learning	Detection of cyber incidents and cyber breaches based on the following modules: firewall, system hardening, secure logging, AI-based anomaly detection and user visualization	Monitoring of physiological parameters

Identification			Expression of need		Application of AI		Performance and purpose	
Industry/ company	**Country**	**Expectation of the solution**	**Expression of the identified need**	**Proposed solution**	**Field and/or means of application of AI**	**Possible techniques and/or actions**	**Alerts and/or features**	**Service rendered in the therapeutic follow-up of the disease**
ARENA2036 eV	Germany	Testing through the cloud to manage the SARS-CoV-2 test	Covid-19 can only be controlled by carrying out thorough testing and immediately responding to known positive cases	Development of a cloud platform (Webservice) with services for the execution of SARS-CoV-2 test procedures and evaluation tools for authorities	Multi-agent systems or distributed artificial intelligence. Signal processing. Machine learning	Deep learning. Multi-agent coordination (multi-agent planning, multi-agent decisions). Distributed problem solving. Searching in a bank of videos and images	Automatic notification of results by telephone message and transmission of laboratory data to authorities	Disease prevention

Identification			Expression of need		Application of AI		Performance and purpose	
Industry/ company	Country	Expectation of the solution	Expression of the identified need	Proposed solution	Field and/or means of application of AI	Possible techniques and/or actions	Alerts and/or features	Service rendered in the therapeutic follow-up of the disease
Lorac Mustaine	Brazil	Artificial intelligence, drones, IoT with sensors and CRISPR	Coronavirus mutations	Use of materials with virus sensors in hospitals to prevent contamination	Robotics. Automatic learning or machine learning. Signal processing and multi-agent systems	Deep learning. Multi-agent coordination (multi-agent planning). Interaction with robots. Bayesian methods. Searching in a video bank	Interactive drones with mechanical arms to carry out patient examinations. Beds with sensors to identify the virus on the spot. Cameras with infrared sensors to identify viruses	Supply chain and detection
Avaamo	United States	Chatbot	The COVID project provides a publicly accessible and interactive Covid-19 intelligent virtual assistant that helps users find information related to the evolution of Covid-19	Construction of a virtual assistant in English with a dialogue box to answer questions or concerns about the coronavirus	Machine learning and human language	Deep learning. Advanced interaction, human language	The virtual assistant ingests millions of pages in real time with systematic updates acquired from the data provided by health authorities	Communication of scientific advice

Identification			Expression of need		Application of AI		Performance and purpose	
Industry/ company	**Country**	**Expectation of the solution**	**Expression of the identified need**	**Proposed solution**	**Field and/or means of application of AI**	**Possible techniques and/or actions**	**Alerts and/or features**	**Service rendered in the therapeutic follow-up of the disease**
ROYBI INC	United States	AI-powered educational robot, distance learning	The robot educates children in language learning and STEM skills. In addition, Roybi Robot helps parents teach at home when schools close during lockdowns	Distance learning, continuing education at home, home schooling, health and safety instructions using a robot	Robotics	Design, perception, decision, action. Interaction with robots. Cognition for robotics and systems	Reports health and safety alerts and encourages children to stay safe and healthy by following the health standards of the competent authorities	Communication of scientific advice
Ezako	France	Automatic detection and prediction of anomalies	Identification of supply anomalies, for example in healthcare facilities	The Upalgo solution helps to automatically provide models that assist in forecasting and detecting anomalies	Automatic learning	Deep learning	/	Supply chain management

Identification			Expression of need		Application of AI		Performance and purpose	
Industry/ company	**Country**	**Expectation of the solution**	**Expression of the identified need**	**Proposed solution**	**Field and/or means of application of AI**	**Possible techniques and/or actions**	**Alerts and/or features**	**Service rendered in the therapeutic follow-up of the disease**
INNOVATION SPRINT SPRL	Belgium	Clinical data management	Facilitating the monitoring of the evolution of symptoms and obtaining information from the system of the measures to be taken, based on an automatic evaluation	The Healthentia app allows individuals to report their health status by answering a simple assessment questionnaire sent to their smartphone	Multi-agent systems	Architecture of the modules that follow on from one other in a predefined order	Automatic notification and monitoring of individuals grouped by the system into potential critical case categories	Detection of sick people
KU Leuven	Belgium	New "human-out" pathogenic laboratory infrastructure	Therapeutics for the treatment of SARS-CoV infection	Drug development focusing on the reuse of existing drugs with the possibility of discovering new agents	Multi-agent systems	Architecture of modules that follow on from one other in a predefined order	/	Medical research on treatments

Identification			Expression of need		Application of AI		Performance and purpose	
Industry/ company	**Country**	**Expectation of the solution**	**Expression of the identified need**	**Proposed solution**	**Field and/or means of application of AI**	**Possible techniques and/or actions**	**Alerts and/or features**	**Service rendered in the therapeutic follow-up of the disease**
Theum AG	Germany	Theum: smart answering machine for the rapid search for knowledge	Search for Covid-19-related knowledge in a rapidly growing ocean of thousands of documents and studies	Theum processes all documentation stored in the cloud or Office 365. The software responds to all user queries with a complete summary of all relevant information in seconds	Machine learning and human language	Deep learning. Advanced interaction, human language	Smart generation of up-to-date Covid-19 documentation from fine granular knowledge networks	Communication of scientific advice

Identification			Expression of need		Application of AI		Performance and purpose	
Industry/ company	Country	Expectation of the solution	Expression of the identified need	Proposed solution	Field and/or means of application of AI	Possible techniques and/or actions	Alerts and/or features	Service rendered in the therapeutic follow-up of the disease
ONHYS	France	ONHYS ONE	The impact of the Covid-19 crisis on essential services is enormous, and it is more necessary than ever for us to make informed decisions and for our leaders to be didactic	ONHYS provides its own simulation of the spread of a virus like Covid-19 in various environments. This solution can be used to optimize flow management when faced with the threat of the spread of a virus and to illustrate the process for the public	Multi-agent systems (agent = software) or distributed artificial intelligence	Multi-agent simulation	The special viral threat module simulates person-to-person and environmental spread for any virus like Covid-19	Detection of sick people
theblue.ai gmbh	Germany	Classification of severe cases based on smartphones	Early detection of severe cases while contributing to meeting the even higher demand for Covid-19 respiratory syndrome diagnostics	Provides diagnostic support on smartphone audio recordings of breath sounds and medical history	Machine learning and human language	Classifier concepts. Supervised learning	The patient is guided through the recording of breath sounds (using the microphone of the smartphone), entering other medical data if available	Telemedicine

Identification			Expression of need		Application of AI		Performance and purpose	
Industry/ company	**Country**	**Expectation of the solution**	**Expression of the identified need**	**Proposed solution**	**Field and/or means of application of AI**	**Possible techniques and/or actions**	**Alerts and/or features**	**Service rendered in the therapeutic follow-up of the disease**
Prenode GmbH	Germany	Scientific data collection Federated automatic learning	/	The MLX system for collecting scientific and distributed data sources of a single type to create robust and superior ML models for a common purpose	Machine learning	Classifier concepts. Regression concepts	Given the sensitive nature of medical data, centralization would be possible based on this system	Communication of scientific advice
AXYN Robotique	France	Telepresence and telemedicine robot	Avoids proximity between patients and health professionals while continuing consultations, diagnoses and medical follow-ups	Ubbo, a remote presence robot that facilitates mobile online video communication between remote people. With its rotating and tilting head, it provides two-way audio/video communication while protecting caregivers	Robotics	Cognition for robotics and systems. Design, perception, decision, action. Interaction with robots	Facilitates a pre-diagnosis by the patient themselves or with the help of a nurse using the Medvir diagnostic application. Reduces the time patients spend in emergency departments and safely regulates incoming patients	Telemedicine

Identification			Expression of need		Application of AI		Performance and purpose	
Industry/ company	Country	Expectation of the solution	Expression of the identified need	Proposed solution	Field and/or means of application of AI	Possible techniques and/or actions	Alerts and/or features	Service rendered in the therapeutic follow-up of the disease
Nobleo Technology	Netherlands	Robots for services in hospitals	Rapid spread of a virus	Construction of a robot to disinfect medical equipment and environments. A complementary software tool is provided, allowing the robot to navigate autonomously and to fully cover the target areas	Robotics. Machine learning	Cognition for robotics and systems. Design, perception, decision, action. Interaction with robots. Bayesian methods. Supervised learning	The robots can disinfect and sterilize areas. The robots can also monitor people's body temperature for early diagnosis	Disinfection

Identification			Expression of need		Application of AI		Performance and purpose	
Industry/ company	**Country**	**Expectation of the solution**	**Expression of the identified need**	**Proposed solution**	**Field and/or means of application of AI**	**Possible techniques and/or actions**	**Alerts and/or features**	**Service rendered in the therapeutic follow-up of the disease**
Swarm Logistics GmbH	Germany	Medical services scheduler/Automatic dispatcher (middleware)	Manual or static planning of circuits and vehicle routes	Software to fully automate the daily dispatch and planning of tour plans, taking into account all constraints (payload, volume, time windows, etc.), as a middleware solution that can be integrated with transport management systems	Machine learning	Deep learning. Advanced interaction, human language. Supervised learning. Latent variables, topical models, causal models and time series	Calculates detailed schedules and trip plans, taking into account constraints. In one mouse click, the user can schedule the route there and back and the pick-up and delivery, calculate the estimated arrival time, calculate the cost of each trip, etc.	Supply chain management

Identification			Expression of need		Application of AI		Performance and purpose	
Industry/ company	Country	Expectation of the solution	Expression of the identified need	Proposed solution	Field and/or means of application of AI	Possible techniques and/or actions	Alerts and/or features	Service rendered in the therapeutic follow-up of the disease
EDI GmbH - Engineering Data Intelligence	Germany	Scientific data collection. Federated machine learning	The main goal of PIBNavi is to control the current pandemic	PIBNavi collects data from various sources to predict the key parameters of the coronavirus pandemic. Specifically tailored to local circumstances, e.g., who to test first, measures that restrict the movement of people, etc.	Machine learning	Deep learning. Supervised learning. Latent variables, topical models, causal models and time series. Predictor concepts	PIBNavi notifies users of their personal risk based on their current behavior, informs users of how their behavior affects the risk of others and helps health authorities take appropriate action	Communication of scientific advice

Identification			Expression of need		Application of AI		Performance and purpose	
Industry/ company	**Country**	**Expectation of the solution**	**Expression of the identified need**	**Proposed solution**	**Field and/or means of application of AI**	**Possible techniques and/or actions**	**Alerts and/or features**	**Service rendered in the therapeutic follow-up of the disease**
Private SME	Serbia	Automated evaluation of the use of protective equipment	In particular, being able to identify locations/areas with high concentrations of people not following recommendations could help EU governments predict potential risk/epidemic locations and act more accurately/locally and in a timely manner instead of constantly warning all countries via mainstream media (which causes negative side effects, including panic)	Development of computer vision algorithms to detect the non-use of personal protective equipment (PPE). Analysis reports would be available as web applications and third party web services	Machine learning	Deep learning. Supervised learning Latent variables, topical models, causal models and time series. Predictor concepts	The solution is designed as a series of successive modules that identify people from images obtained from surveillance/IP/USB cameras, then inspect whether that person is wearing a mask, gloves, etc.	Communication of scientific advice

Identification			Expression of need		Application of AI		Performance and purpose	
Industry/ company	Country	Expectation of the solution	Expression of the identified need	Proposed solution	Field and/or means of application of AI	Possible techniques and/or actions	Alerts and/or features	Service rendered in the therapeutic follow-up of the disease
PAL Robotics	Spain	Robot for hospital services	Hospitals face logistical challenges beyond crisis situations. Moving around the hospital to deliver medications, documents or blood samples takes a lot of time for every caregiver and nurse while also putting them at risk of infection	TIAGo Delivery is a solution capable of transporting various objects such as medicines, samples or food, in hospitals or similar environments. It can be extended with features such as thermal cameras or other health monitoring devices, helping caregivers on the front line	Autonomous robotics and signal processing	Cognition for robotics and systems. Design, perception, decision, action. Interaction with robots. Bayesian methods. Supervised learning. Activity recognition	The autonomous robot quickly and safely delivers the various items needed, minimizing social interaction and and the spread of infections thanks to its organized configuration in shelves. It is constantly aware of any changes and the presence of obstacles (people or machines) thanks to the integrated sensors, which guarantee safety and efficiency	Supply chain management

Identification			Expression of need		Application of AI		Performance and purpose	
Industry/ company	Country	Expectation of the solution	Expression of the identified need	Proposed solution	Field and/or means of application of AI	Possible techniques and/or actions	Alerts and/or features	Service rendered in the therapeutic follow-up of the disease
PAL Robotics	Spain	Service robots in hospitals (assistance for and monitoring of patients)	This solution addresses at least two main issues facing hospitals and institutions: – the lack of optimization of hospital first aid, especially when healthcare professionals are overly exposed to potentially ill users with insufficient protection or resources; – the widespread quarantine of users also results in the prolonged isolation of individuals from social interactions, which can have a negative impact on mental health	PAL Robotics' humanoid social robot ARI functions as a hospital receptionist, helping to clarify general queries and control the flow of new incoming users. It also provides monitoring and assistance to users affected by Covid-19, for example, who need to be isolated	Autonomous robotics and signal processing	Cognition for robotics and systems. Design, perception, decision, action. Interaction with robots. Bayesian methods. Supervised learning. Activity recognition. Speech recognition and and machine translation	The ARI social robot could be teleoperated and maintain ongoing social interactions and adherence to treatment regimens without fear of spreading disease. The robot can be upgraded with additional features	Telemedicine

Identification			Expression of need		Application of AI		Performance and purpose	
Industry/ company	**Country**	**Expectation of the solution**	**Expression of the identified need**	**Proposed solution**	**Field and/or means of application of AI**	**Possible techniques and/or actions**	**Alerts and/or features**	**Service rendered in the therapeutic follow-up of the disease**
IM-COVID19	Spain	Medical imaging	/	Covid-19 diagnosis using medical images applying artificial intelligence to identify itself as a prefilter	Machine learning	Deep learning. Supervised learning. Latent variables, topical models, causal models and time series. Predictor concepts	Diagnosis based on biomedical images	Telemedicine

Identification			Expression of need		Application of AI		Performance and purpose	
Industry/ company	Country	Expectation of the solution	Expression of the identified need	Proposed solution	Field and/or means of application of AI	Possible techniques and/or actions	Alerts and/or features	Service rendered in the therapeutic follow-up of the disease
apoQlar GmbH	Germany	VSI Holomedicine Pandemic Package	Only selected physicians conduct patient visits and admissions to protect other physicians from infection. These physicians can consult with their colleagues at any time, regardless of their location, if they have questions or doubts. This can also be applied to the emergency room to maintain emergency care	If the doctor/assistant on site has questions, they can call a colleague or specialist through the VSI Holomedicine glasses. The holograms appear as 3D objects in space and are perceived through suitable glasses, such as the Microsoft HoloLens. The called colleague receives the exact field of view of the caller on their laptop or smartphone and can advise them optimally without being on site themselves	Machine learning. Mixed reality. Virtual reality. Augmented virtual reality	Deep learning. Supervised learning. Latent variables, topical models, causal models and time series. Predictor concepts	Doctors can collaborate through the connected glasses. The other side sees what the doctors see, including a hologram with quick documentation, as well as text dictation, photos and video recordings, which are automatically recorded by citodensitometry: Covid-19 detection in CT images rendered in 3D in mixed reality	Telemedicine

Identification			Expression of need		Application of AI		Performance and purpose	
Industry/ company	Country	Expectation of the solution	Expression of the identified need	Proposed solution	Field and/or means of application of AI	Possible techniques and/or actions	Alerts and/or features	Service rendered in the therapeutic follow-up of the disease
Novadécouverte	France	Nova Covid-19 knowledge-based model	The search for a vaccine and a treatment has become a top priority in the fight against Covid-19 and its multiple variants. The search for a specific drug for this virus is fraught with difficulties despite the efforts of scientific researchers around the world. The question of which drug to develop among the hundreds of molecules available to provide an optimal response to this virus remains open	Knowledge-based technology platform based on a multi-scale and multi-level mathematical model of the Covid-19 disease, integrating the virus, its target cells, the immune system and the organs involved (lungs, kidneys, intestines), the individuals and the population in which they have social interactions	Multi-agent systems (agent = software) or distributed artificial intelligence	Multi-agent simulation	Exploration and platform selection based on the clinical benefit of novel therapeutic/ preventive approaches, including combinations, the optimization of in vitro/in vivo experiments and clinical trials, the optimization of therapeutic regimens and the shortening of clinical development	Medical research for a treatment

Identification			Expression of need		Application of AI		Performance and purpose	
Industry/ company	**Country**	**Expectation of the solution**	**Expression of the identified need**	**Proposed solution**	**Field and/or means of application of AI**	**Possible techniques and/or actions**	**Alerts and/or features**	**Service rendered in the therapeutic follow-up of the disease**
BlueBright	Belgium	Chatbot	Many people are still spamming forums and social networks about Covid-19. Fake news is spreading and hospital call centers are exploding	Providing key answers for Covid-19 and also the ability to be routed to the local telemedicine network	Multi-agent systems (agent = software)	Multi-agent simulation	FAQ chatbot, robot chatbot trends, psychological support chatbot	Telemedicine
Bournemouth University	United Kingdom	AI remote diagnoses of patients' respiratory health	Europe has a large number of citizens with chronic obstructive pulmonary disease (COPD) and other respiratory diseases. This is one of the high-risk groups that may be exposed to Covid-19. This is also true for elderly people with underlying cardiovascular diseases	Automated method for detecting symptoms of breathing difficulties in Covid-19 infected individuals	Machine learning	Deep learning. Supervised learning. Latent variables, topical models, causal models and time series. Classifier concepts. Data mining	Individuals in the home give consent to access their respiratory audio data and geolocations. The data are transmitted with their respective diagnoses to health-care staff with real-time map identification of infected population segments	Detection of sick people

Identification			Expression of need		Application of AI		Performance and purpose	
Industry/ company	Country	Expectation of the solution	Expression of the identified need	Proposed solution	Field and/or means of application of AI	Possible techniques and/or actions	Alerts and/or features	Service rendered in the therapeutic follow-up of the disease
Factorisation (delayed start-up due to the impact of Covid-19 on the industry)	Netherlands	Service robot	The rapidly changing environment is pushing healthcare systems to automate, digitally transform and continuously adapt. Healthcare experts need a fast and agile way to create new and digital solutions. The lack of coding and automation expertise is pushing these tasks onto IT experts who lack domain knowledge and are not widely available	Factorise Edge provides plug-and-play connectivity for robots (and other devices) and seamlessly connects hardware to Siemens' low-code rapid application development platform Mendix. Factorise Edge extends this approach to automation and robotics solutions	Robotization. Multi-agent systems (agent = software) or distributed artificial intelligence. Signal processing. Machine learning	Deep learning. Supervised learning. Latent variables, topical models, causal models and time series. Multi-agent simulation	In Mendix, domain experts can create complete user interfaces and occupational approaches by integrating them into mobile devices and web platforms. Devices (robot arms, measurement devices, scanners) can be connected to the Factorise Edge box. Map device functionality via pre-configured mapping to a low-code environment	Telemedicine

Identification			Expression of need		Application of AI		Performance and purpose	
Industry/ company	Country	Expectation of the solution	Expression of the identified need	Proposed solution	Field and/or means of application of AI	Possible techniques and/or actions	Alerts and/or features	Service rendered in the therapeutic follow-up of the disease
BigML Labs, SAU	Spain	Diagnostic platform	Anomaly detection, early diagnosis, triage, demand forecasting, personalized treatments and many other predictive use cases	Platform that accelerates the development of end-to-end data-driven applications	Machine learning	Deep learning. Supervised learning. Latent variables, topical models, causal models and time series	BigML's unparalleled interpretability, explainability, traceability and reproducibility, which are implemented at the core, can help users to make better data-driven decisions and automate a number of critical tasks to combat the current pandemic and anticipate new ones	Detection of sick people

Identification			Expression of need		Application of AI		Performance and purpose	
Industry/ company	Country	Expectation of the solution	Expression of the identified need	Proposed solution	Field and/or means of application of AI	Possible techniques and/or actions	Alerts and/or features	Service rendered in the therapeutic follow-up of the disease
Softbrik	Estonia	Consultation platform	91% of Europeans under the age of 50 have one health check-up every 25 months. This makes early detection and rapid containment of any communicable disease impossible with an average of 3.2 doctors per 1,000 inhabitants across the continent	Softbrik reinvents the home doctor in the digital age with a remote consultation platform. Softbrik's algorithms detect Covid-19 keywords, select symptoms such as "I have a dry cough" and alert doctors in order of priority to take immediate action	Machine learning	Deep learning. Supervised learning. Latent variables, topical models, causal models and time series	Healthcare professionals remotely create their account in 10 minutes and send the link/SMS to their existing or potential patient households. Patients can communicate to provide information about their health. Sharing languages available: English, Italian, Spanish, German and French. Softbrik provides physicians with voice files for further analysis	Telemedicine

Identification			Expression of need		Application of AI		Performance and purpose	
Industry/ company	**Country**	**Expectation of the solution**	**Expression of the identified need**	**Proposed solution**	**Field and/or means of application of AI**	**Possible techniques and/or actions**	**Alerts and/or features**	**Service rendered in the therapeutic follow-up of the disease**
Robotics and training services in Ireland	Ireland	Hazardous waste removal in hospitals and sterilization	Potential contact with hazardous waste and non-sterile surfaces	Manual	Robotics. Machine learning	Deep learning. Supervised learning. Latent variables, topical models, causal models and time series. Cognition for robotics and systems. Design, perception, decision, action	Using AIV to move bins and using UV light. The AIV used can move 90–1000 kg	Disinfection

Identification			Expression of need		Application of AI		Performance and purpose	
Industry/ company	**Country**	**Expectation of the solution**	**Expression of the identified need**	**Proposed solution**	**Field and/or means of application of AI**	**Possible techniques and/or actions**	**Alerts and/or features**	**Service rendered in the therapeutic follow-up of the disease**
E.ON Digital Technology/ Stanford University	Germany	AI-based handwashing coach	Regular and proper handwashing is essential to slowing and eventually stopping the spread of Covid-19. However, most people do not know how to wash their hands properly, even if they do it regularly	Deep learning-based solution that analyzes videos of people washing their hands and gives immediate feedback to the handwashing user on how to do better	Machine learning. Signal processing	Deep learning. Supervised learning. Latent variables, topical models, causal models and time series. Activity recognition. Searching in an image database. Searching in a video database	By installing cameras on sinks, for example in restrooms in restaurants, kindergartens, museums, public restrooms, etc., the system can evaluate videos of people washing their hands and give visual or audio feedback on how to improve their handwashing habits	Disinfection

Identification			Expression of need		Application of AI		Performance and purpose	
Industry/ company	Country	Expectation of the solution	Expression of the identified need	Proposed solution	Field and/or means of application of AI	Possible techniques and/or actions	Alerts and/or features	Service rendered in the therapeutic follow-up of the disease
Independent	Spain	Askcovid	The need for accurate and reliable information on Covid-19. There is a growing urgency for these approaches due to the rapid acceleration of new literature on coronaviruses, making it difficult for medical research to keep pace	Developing a textual data mining tool to help the medical community develop answers to priority scientific questions. Querying questions in a database of over 900 scientific studies on Covid-19 and obtaining an accurate answer using artificial intelligence	Natural language processing and machine learning	Multi-agent systems (agent = software) or distributed artificial intelligence	The solution provides a fast and accurate method to access scientific information on Covid-19. The database consists of more than 33,000 full-text scientific articles on Covid-19, SARS-CoV-2 and related coronaviruses	Communication of scientific advice

Identification			Expression of need		Application of AI		Performance and purpose	
Industry/ company	Country	Expectation of the solution	Expression of the identified need	Proposed solution	Field and/or means of application of AI	Possible techniques and/or actions	Alerts and/or features	Service rendered in the therapeutic follow-up of the disease
University of Oslo	Norway	DHIS2	Collection and dissemination of epidemic data from each health facility	Data on individual cases, contacts and arrivals, as well as aggregated information (figures). Customized configuration packages have been developed for the DHIS2 platform, which is a national health management information system present in more than 60 countries	Natural language processing and machine learning. Multi-agent systems (agent = software) or distributed artificial intelligence	Deep learning. Supervised learning. Latent variables, topical models, causal models and time series	With DHIS2, Covid-19 packages can be used support surveillance workflows and the automated analysis of key components of routine and active surveillance. It enrolls and tracks suspected cases; captures symptoms, demographics, risk factors and exposures; creates laboratory requests; links confirmed cases to contacts; and monitors patient outcomes	Monitoring of physiological parameters

Identification			Expression of need		Application of AI		Performance and purpose	
Industry/ company	Country	Expectation of the solution	Expression of the identified need	Proposed solution	Field and/or means of application of AI	Possible techniques and/or actions	Alerts and/or features	Service rendered in the therapeutic follow-up of the disease
Fintricity	United Kingdom	Kendra Labs	AI	A data/AI platform that allows data to be aggregated and then processed quickly. The framework and open source platform were created by Inte	Natural language processing and machine learning. Multi-agent systems (agent = software) or distributed artificial intelligence	Deep learning. Supervised learning. Latent variables, topical models, causal models and time series	Collects data and enables data scientists to process, match and model them	Communication of scientific advice

Identification			Expression of need		Application of AI		Performance and purpose	
Industry/ company	**Country**	**Expectation of the solution**	**Expression of the identified need**	**Proposed solution**	**Field and/or means of application of AI**	**Possible techniques and/or actions**	**Alerts and/or features**	**Service rendered in the therapeutic follow-up of the disease**
PAL Robotics	Spain	Autonomous disinfection robot (ADR) that uses UV-C lamps	Cleaning and disinfection activities in hospitals and institutions are performed manually and some areas must be disinfected after each use (e.g., when a room is cleaned and prepared for the next patient). Manual disinfection carries the risk of spreading infections rather than cleaning contaminated surfaces	A disinfection robot is an autonomous solution capable of performing cleaning and disinfection in hospitals and medical centers	Robotics. Machine learning	Deep learning. Supervised learning. Latent variables, topical models, causal models and time series. Cognition for robotics and systems. Design, perception, decision, action	ADRs navigate autonomously in an environment, finding the best route to ensure the disinfection of the whole space with UV-C lamps, and are constantly aware of any change thanks to the integrated sensors, which guarantee safety and efficiency	Disinfection

Identification			Expression of need		Application of AI		Performance and purpose	
Industry/ company	Country	Expectation of the solution	Expression of the identified need	Proposed solution	Field and/or means of application of AI	Possible techniques and/or actions	Alerts and/or features	Service rendered in the therapeutic follow-up of the disease
ROBO. AI GmbH	Germany	Cosibot, a "Stay informed" Covid-19 robot	Citizens across Europe receive daily updates from all media. Much of this information is often fragmented, contradictory and biased	Cosibot offers all the answers on coronavirus to EU populations with qualified information from official sources in one place and it can be customized for each country. Cosibot allows written and oral interaction, enabling people with visual and hearing impairments to access the information	Robotics. Machine learning	Deep learning. Supervised learning. Latent variables, topical models, causal models and time series. Cognition for robotics and systems. Design, perception, decision, action	It provides information to government organizations to gauge public sentiment. Cosibot is multilingual and available 24/7. It is multi-channel, accessible by voice, web and all social media tools	Communication of scientific advice

Identification			Expression of need		Application of AI		Performance and purpose	
Industry/ company	Country	Expectation of the solution	Expression of the identified need	Proposed solution	Field and/or means of application of AI	Possible techniques and/or actions	Alerts and/or features	Service rendered in the therapeutic follow-up of the disease
Kadima BV	Netherlands	Covid-19 risk assessment and monitoring platform	The need to have updated information on best practices to fight the virus. The need for information on health measures announced by government authorities to eradicate the virus	From the information collected with this solution, it is possible to assign patients who must be seen immediately by a healthcare professional and also reduce the pressure on tests/hospitalization	Machine learning	Deep learning. Supervised learning. Latent variables, topical models, causal models and time series	The solution includes the remote monitoring of patient progress, automated patient queries, alerts to providers about high-risk patients, and daily updates on community/regional disease transmission and spread	Detection of sick people

Identification			Expression of need		Application of AI		Performance and purpose	
Industry/ company	Country	Expectation of the solution	Expression of the identified need	Proposed solution	Field and/or means of application of AI	Possible techniques and/or actions	Alerts and/or features	Service rendered in the therapeutic follow-up of the disease
BBZ srl	Italy	LEO console for remote operation	The LEO console solves the problem of operator safety when handling or moving infected equipment in hazardous environments. The LEO console, in fact, can be used to control any remote operation device, fixed or mobile, from a remote and secure location	A teleoperation platform can be developed by integrating existing robotic handling platforms with the LEO console. The console can be integrated with several robotic arms	Robotics. Machine learning	Deep learning. Supervised learning. Latent variables, topical models, causal models and time series. Cognition for robotics and systems. Design, perception, decision, action	The LEO console is a lightweight, portable teleoperation console consisting of a stereoscopic vision system, two 7DOF input devices and a footswitch. The console provides a high definition stereoscopic view of the remote scene and two input devices	Detection of sick people

Identification			Expression of need		Application of AI		Performance and purpose	
Industry/ company	Country	Expectation of the solution	Expression of the identified need	Proposed solution	Field and/or means of application of AI	Possible techniques and/or actions	Alerts and/or features	Service rendered in the therapeutic follow-up of the disease
DARVIS Health	Germany	DARVIS healthcare hygiene solution	PPE clothing and hand hygiene are the primary protective measures against infection for healthcare workers and patients. The health and associated operational capacity of healthcare workers, physicians and emergency departments in their clinics is a valuable factor in the fight against coronavirus. Crisis situations, massive stress and long working hours result in unintentional errors in the correct and vital use of protective clothing and necessary hand hygiene	Instant feedback is provided based on hand disinfection or the correct wearing of PPE clothing. The solution is based on a computer vision platform that has already been deployed in a clinic in Hanover for inventory tracking and has been adjusted for this use case	Machine learning	Deep learning. Supervised learning. Latent variables, topical models, causal models and time series	Digitally determines at the access barriers of the hygiene areas whether protective clothing (surgical gowns, gloves, masks) is being worn correctly	Disinfection

Identification			Expression of need		Application of AI		Performance and purpose	
Industry/ company	Country	Expectation of the solution	Expression of the identified need	Proposed solution	Field and/or means of application of AI	Possible techniques and/or actions	Alerts and/or features	Service rendered in the therapeutic follow-up of the disease
OXIFRAME SL	Spain	CORONAZERO	Authorities are not able to identify symptoms or asymptomatic or early cases for infected individuals prior to any call made to the health services or the Public Safety Answering Point (PSAP)/112	CORONAZERO is an online software tool based on the self-assessment of symptoms and a real-time contagion probability tool for any individual	Machine learning	Predictor concepts. Deep learning. Supervised learning. Latent variables, topical models, causal models and time series	An online survey that collects anonymous and mass information on infectiousness and symptoms to locate outbreaks of asymptomatic people. CORONAZERO is an AI-based GIS tool that locates areas of infection and predicts contagion risks geographically	Prediction of disease progression
Methinks Software	Spain	MethinksCOVID	Methinks aims to create a diagnostic tool to predict the outcome of Covid-19 patients in crisis	The Methinks tool allows you to enter a chest X-ray and basic clinical data and will display the probability in the next 24/48 hours of the need for hospitalization or intensive care	Machine learning	Predictor concepts. Deep learning. Supervised learning. Latent variables, topical models, causal models and time series	The diagnosis of Covid-19 can be made by any means, including PCR testing, medical imaging or even just the clinical symptoms. The probability is calculated and the result is given after 24/48h indicating the need for hospitalization or not	Prediction of disease progression

Identification			Expression of need		Application of AI		Performance and purpose	
Industry/ company	Country	Expectation of the solution	Expression of the identified need	Proposed solution	Field and/or means of application of AI	Possible techniques and/or actions	Alerts and/or features	Service rendered in the therapeutic follow-up of the disease
Shark Robotics	France	RHYNO PROTECT disinfecting robot	**Shark Robotics** decided to create the Rhyno Protect disinfecting decontamination robot. Operated remotely, this robot fights against the virus without exposing humans while keeping them away from possible contamination	The robot is designed to disinfect the surfaces of living spaces by micro-spraying disinfectant liquid and to decontaminate the ambient air by killing airborne pathogenic micro-organisms using the UV-C lamp	Robotics	Cognition for robotics and systems. Design, perception, decision, action	It can destroy pathogenic micro-organisms present in the air thanks to UV-C lamps (internationally patented system)	Disinfection
Innovation management Sinfonic Bt	Hungary	Digital saliva test	Each virus functions differently in the body, stimulating a different immunological profile, and the high concentration of Covid-19 virus in saliva can affect the structure of saliva	Early warning system before hospitalization to support Covid-19 research by comparing saliva samples from Covid-19 patients to a database with samples from a healthy population	Natural language processing and machine learning. Multi-agent systems (agent = software) or distributed artificial intelligence	Deep learning. Supervised learning. Latent variables, topical models, causal models and time series. Searching in an image bank	This system works using an online computer vision algorithm to detect saliva crystals for ovulation prediction in images of samples taken by mobile devices. This algorithm is trained from a database of thousands of images of dried saliva samples from a healthy population	Monitoring of physiological parameters

Identification			Expression of need		Application of AI		Performance and purpose	
Industry/ company	**Country**	**Expectation of the solution**	**Expression of the identified need**	**Proposed solution**	**Field and/or means of application of AI**	**Possible techniques and/or actions**	**Alerts and/or features**	**Service rendered in the therapeutic follow-up of the disease**
ContentWise BVBA	Belgium	Tooly.Bot	Advanced remote care for the patient at home, telepresence, relieving medical staff by automating tedious tasks in a generic way. Automation of a portable mini-laboratory	Tooly is a low-cost wearable robot equipped with 3D vision that can automate tedious tasks such as sample collection, patient monitoring with AI detection of breathing from posture and chest movements, cough detection, bleeding, and fall detection	Machine learning and human language. Natural language processing. Signal processing	Deep learning. Supervised learning. Latent variables, topical models, causal models and time series. Searching in an image bank. Object tracking and motion analysis	The robot has five degrees of freedom, 3D vision and an IR sensor, and AI vision recognition. It can run on batteries or aUSB-C power source. The robot does not store images but only extracts meanings, ensuring that privacy is respected	Telemedicine

Identification			Expression of need		Application of AI		Performance and purpose	
Industry/ company	Country	Expectation of the solution	Expression of the identified need	Proposed solution	Field and/or means of application of AI	Possible techniques and/or actions	Alerts and/or features	Service rendered in the therapeutic follow-up of the disease
OMQ + Userlike	Germany	CoronAssist Bot. Interactive information system for FAQs	People have many questions about symptoms, behaviors, prophylactic measures, their own illnesses, the number of cases and risk assessment, among other urgent questions about the current situation. Institutions are completely overwhelmed by the volume of questions and lack the staff to answer	Building a chatbot that can access other knowledge sources effortlessly. The chatbot engages in dialogue	Machine learning and human language. Processing of natural language Signal processing	Deep learning. Supervised learning. Latent variables, topical models, causal models and time series. Searching in an image bank. Object tracking and motion analysis	The questions and answers are stored in the central knowledge base. The service is rendered in the therapeutic follow-up of Covid-19. Available in several European languages and on several channels (website, WhatsApp, SMS, etc.)	Communication of scientific advice

Identification			Expression of need		Application of AI		Performance and purpose	
Industry/ company	**Country**	**Expectation of the solution**	**Expression of the identified need**	**Proposed solution**	**Field and/or means of application of AI**	**Possible techniques and/or actions**	**Alerts and/or features**	**Service rendered in the therapeutic follow-up of the disease**
Findest	Netherlands	Launch of the free COVID-19 technology search engine, IGOR ^ COV19	While companies and researchers are working day and night, it may be that the solutions to the sub-challenges of beating Covid-19 already exist – perhaps at a university, in a completely different industry or having been invented last week by a company	The IGOR AI solution has been temporarily transformed into IGOR ^ COV19 and will be freely available for all scientists and R&D professionals to use to find technologies that will help them innovate around the challenges posed by Covid-19	Multi-agent systems (agent = software) or distributed artificial intelligence. Machine learning	Deep learning. Supervised learning. Latent variables, topical models, causal models and time series. Multi-agent learning (language, platforms)	IGOR AI is built as a functional technology search engine. IGOR ^ COV19 is the edition specifically designed for functional searches such as "coronavirus test"	Communication of scientific advice

Identification			Expression of need		Application of AI		Performance and purpose	
Industry/company	Country	Expectation of the solution	Expression of the identified need	Proposed solution	Field and/or means of application of AI	Possible techniques and/or actions	Alerts and/or features	Service rendered in the therapeutic follow-up of the disease
UiPath	Romania	UiPath RPA platform	Employee health screening (could be used for hospital staff) and isolated individuals. Efficiency: automate operational processes (e.g. streamline the supply chain by determining the optimal inventory according to the context). Search robot: fast online search	Robot platforms that use the user interface to capture data and manipulate applications as humans do. They can be used by healthcare professionals. For example, nurses spend hours inputting test results into systems, which can be done by robots	Robotics. Natural language processing. Signal processing. Multi-agent systems (agent = software) or distributed artificial intelligence	Cognition for robotics and systems. Design, perception, decision, action. Searching in an image bank. Object tracking and motion analysis. Multi-agent learning (language, platforms)	Software bots emulate and integrate the actions of a human interacting in digital systems to execute a business process. Covid-19 test acceleration capability. Formal question and answer bots	Communication of scientific advice

Identification			Expression of need		Application of AI		Performance and purpose	
Industry/ company	**Country**	**Expectation of the solution**	**Expression of the identified need**	**Proposed solution**	**Field and/or means of application of AI**	**Possible techniques and/or actions**	**Alerts and/or features**	**Service rendered in the therapeutic follow-up of the disease**
SuccessData	United Kingdom	Automating the extraction of research/ diagnostic information	The SuccessData platform will showcase the latest developments in AI research around text and data mining approaches to finding answers to questions and connecting information about that content in support of ongoing Covid-19 response efforts around the world	The SuccessData platform will showcase the latest developments in AI research around text and data mining approaches to finding answers to questions	Multi-agent systems (agent = software) or distributed artificial intelligence. Machine learning	Deep learning. Supervised learning. Latent variables, topical models, causal models and time series	SuccessData can systematically extract, streamline and standardize information from the growing body of medical research on Covid-19, SARS-CoV-2 and related coronaviruses to facilitate and accelerate downstream analysis by researchers	Communication of scientific advice

Identification			Expression of need		Application of AI		Performance and purpose	
Industry/ company	Country	Expectation of the solution	Expression of the identified need	Proposed solution	Field and/or means of application of AI	Possible techniques and/or actions	Alerts and/or features	Service rendered in the therapeutic follow-up of the disease
Synergy Management Consulting Cyprus Ltd	Cyprus	BIOLAB 360	Health telematics, remote healthcare	A health app that can remotely monitor a patient's vital signals 24 hours a day and receive remote alerts in real time	Neuroscience, cognitive science. Machine learning	Understanding deep learning. Supervised learning. Latent variables, topical models, causal models and time series	The system supports automated measurements of patients' vital signs. These measurements are automated via a secure Bluetooth protocol in the tablet software application and the measurement data is automatically replicated in the cloud and sent to the corresponding physician, hospital or remote Medical Call Center application (app or online)	Telemedicine

Identification			Expression of need		Application of AI		Performance and purpose	
Industry/ company	**Country**	**Expectation of the solution**	**Expression of the identified need**	**Proposed solution**	**Field and/or means of application of AI**	**Possible techniques and/or actions**	**Alerts and/or features**	**Service rendered in the therapeutic follow-up of the disease**
Solteq Plc	Finland	Autonomous telepresence robot for hospitals	Reducing the risk of personnel contamination and consumption of protective equipment by using the remote capabilities of Solteq's existing robotics platform from the retail robotics solution. Solteq's retail robot is a proven stand-alone solution	An autonomous and/or remote-controlled robot can bring telecommunication and diagnostic tools into the restricted area and staff can remotely check conditions and communicate with the patient	Robotics. Natural language processing. Signal processing. Multi-agent systems (agent = software) or distributed artificial intelligence	Cognition for robotics and systems. Design, perception, decision, action. Searching in an image bank. Object tracking and motion analysis. Multi-agent learning (language, platforms)	More than 10 hours of autonomy with a single charge. Can support a load of 100 kg. Customizable with different containers, sensors and equipment. Autonomous/remote control driving, telepresence functionality, UV disinfection, remote temperature measurements, patient pulse measurements and oxygen saturation measurements	Disinfection

Identification			Expression of need		Application of AI		Performance and purpose	
Industry/ company	Country	Expectation of the solution	Expression of the identified need	Proposed solution	Field and/or means of application of AI	Possible techniques and/or actions	Alerts and/or features	Service rendered in the therapeutic follow-up of the disease
eHidra	Spain	Contact tracer	Following and advising people who have been in close contact with an infected person, as validated by a doctor. This should then prove that two people have been in contact. The processes of testing scans and advertising in peripheral cycles still need to be improved. The results are stored in an SQLite database integrated in the application	Application on Android and iOS, for which you can register using your phone number. Registration data are stored in Firebase (Google servers) and are therefore fully scalable	Multi-agent systems (agent = software) or distributed artificial intelligence	Object tracking and motion analysis. Multi-agent learning	All data are encrypted and stored in a local database that will only be used in case of infection to analyze the data and inform people who might be infected. The point of the application is to be able to recognize and connect to other devices, regardless of the platform, and to exchange information. This will facilitate contact tracing	Detection of sick people

Identification			Expression of need		Application of AI		Performance and purpose	
Industry/ company	**Country**	**Expectation of the solution**	**Expression of the identified need**	**Proposed solution**	**Field and/or means of application of AI**	**Possible techniques and/or actions**	**Alerts and/or features**	**Service rendered in the therapeutic follow-up of the disease**
UEM	Spain	Defense architecture for patient monitoring via AI and the IoT	Remote patient care	Through the integration of AI, the IoT (tested and certified devices) and blockchain	Multi-agent systems (agent = software) or distributed artificial intelligence	Object tracking and motion analysis. Multi-agent learning	Measurement of oxygen levels, blood pressure, temperature. Remote alarm management by physicians or a caregiver, with an intuitive panel, patient history, etc. Real-time monitoring	Detection of sick people
OPT/NET BV	Netherlands	OptOSS AI	The enforcement of quarantine measures and the rapid follow-up of infected people who are contagious is essential in the early stages of any pandemic	OptOSS AI is capable of processing huge amounts of mobile network logs on the activity of all connected devices (e.g., cell phones). This OPT/NET product provides an application for health agencies to monitor the location of infected individuals or track their past locations	Multi-agent systems (agent = software) or distributed artificial intelligence. Machine learning	Deep learning. Supervised learning. Latent variables, topical models, causal models and time series	Measurement of oxygen levels, blood pressure, temperature. Remote alarm management by physicians or a caregiver, with an intuitive panel, patient history, etc. Real-time monitoring	Monitoring of physiological parameters

Identification			Expression of need		Application of AI		Performance and purpose	
Industry/ company	**Country**	**Expectation of the solution**	**Expression of the identified need**	**Proposed solution**	**Field and/or means of application of AI**	**Possible techniques and/or actions**	**Alerts and/or features**	**Service rendered in the therapeutic follow-up of the disease**
Czech Technical University in Prague	Czech Republic/ Prague	Recommendations for essential travel times using crowd prediction	The central idea of the project is to minimize people's potential exposure to infection by advising them to plan their necessary travel in consideration of the expected density of other people at the site	A community data collection application that assesses the density and number of people in exposed locations (stores, parks, hospitals, etc.) and sends anonymous data to a server that performs a forecast of the day using spatio-temporal models such as FreMEn	Multi-agent systems (agent = software) or distributed artificial intelligence	Object tracking and motion analysis. Multi-agent learning	Spatio-temporal models that can predict future densities of people in various locations with epidemiological models, which can estimate transmission and exposure risks	Detection of sick people
Rulex Innovations Labs Srl	Italy	Optimization of the supply chain with Rulex Analytics software	One of the major challenges of Covid-19 management is to optimize the supply chain in healthcare centers	The proposed solution aims to optimize the supply chain by ensuring the right level of procurement for both raw materials and medical devices	Machine learning to calculate optimal movements in the network and make them available to other systems	Understanding. Deep learning. Supervised learning. Latent variables, topical models, causal models and time series	The solution is designed to ensure resilience (the system can provide a sub-optimal solution even in critical situations), rapid deployment (it only needs to be connected to the right data sources) and adaptability (it automatically adapts to rapidly changing situations)	Supply chain management

Identification			Expression of need		Application of AI		Performance and purpose	
Industry/ company	Country	Expectation of the solution	Expression of the identified need	Proposed solution	Field and/or means of application of AI	Possible techniques and/or actions	Alerts and/or features	Service rendered in the therapeutic follow-up of the disease
Han's Robot Germany GmbH	Germany	AI-based contactless health and motion monitoring system	In order to monitor the main vital parameters of humans (pulse, respiratory rate and temperature), special equipment is usually required	Integrated monitoring systems capable of identifying the vital parameters of several people in a room at the same time. In addition, people's movements, as well as the current position of a person's body in the room, can be detected while completely protecting their privacy, and the data can be viewed locally or remotely	Machine learning. Signal processing	Understanding. Deep learning. Supervised learning. Latent variables, topical models, causal models and time series. Object tracking and motion analysis	These sensor systems use a combination of high-precision radio frequency and infrared measurements to determine a point cloud of highly accurate position, temperature and velocity information	Detection of sick people

Identification			Expression of need		Application of AI		Performance and purpose	
Industry/ company	Country	Expectation of the solution	Expression of the identified need	Proposed solution	Field and/or means of application of AI	Possible techniques and/or actions	Alerts and/or features	Service rendered in the therapeutic follow-up of the disease
EPOS Health Management	Germany	mycare2x	Admitting a patient with a pre-existing multilingual electronic medical record (EMR) to support hospitals with online paperless multilingual EMRs; cloud backup for scientific analysis and international medical cooperation via telemedicine with an artificial intelligence (AI) interface for diagnostic support	The multilingual EMR with GPS tracker is web-based and Open Source, can be pre-filled by individuals at home and gives feedback based on the condition. On admission, the EMR is already available to hospital staff. For example, pneumothorax, cardiomegaly, enlarged cardio mediastinum, etc.	Machine learning to aid diagnosis using X-ray/medical imaging of suspected Covid cases	Understanding. Deep learning. Supervised learning. Latent variables, topical models, causal models and time series. Object tracking and motion analysis	Individuals can enter data from home, patients can be geolocated and medical staff can continue to use the EMR in hospitals seamlessly when individuals are admitted. It has full telemedicine functionality and an AI interface, as well as an interface for other AI diagnostic functions	Telemedicine

Identification			Expression of need		Application of AI		Performance and purpose	
Industry/ company	**Country**	**Expectation of the solution**	**Expression of the identified need**	**Proposed solution**	**Field and/or means of application of AI**	**Possible techniques and/or actions**	**Alerts and/or features**	**Service rendered in the therapeutic follow-up of the disease**
FLUIDDA NV	United States	AI predicting which Covid-19 patients will require intensive care	This model predicts which patients will eventually require intensive care (oxygenation/ ventilation) after testing positive for Covid-19	The primary functionality of this model is to predict whether new Covid-19 patients will eventually require ICU management with ventilation/ oxygenation to ensure their survival	Machine learning. Signal processing	Understanding. Deep learning trained on a set of existing CT scans. Predictor concepts. Supervised learning. Latent variables, topical models, causal models and time series. Object tracking and motion analysis	Adequate data from new patients testing positive for Covid-19 will be evaluated by a model to predict whether that patient will eventually require intensive care. This will be undertaken by analyzing a simple CT scan	Detection of sick people

Identification			Expression of need		Application of AI		Performance and purpose	
Industry/company	Country	Expectation of the solution	Expression of the identified need	Proposed solution	Field and/or means of application of AI	Possible techniques and/or actions	Alerts and/or features	Service rendered in the therapeutic follow-up of the disease
Ternow AI	Germany	Automatic Covid-19 diagnosis powered by AI using visual data	Rapid diagnosis of Covid-19: rapidly separating infected individuals is the primary and most effective response to an outbreak. This is achieved by inspecting medical CT images, X-ray sensors or thermal imaging cameras or microscopic blood sample images and by inspecting individuals or a large group of people passing in front of the camera	The AI-powered algorithm is intended for Covid-19 diagnosis	Machine learning. Signal processing	Understanding. Deep learning that will be trained on a set of existing. CT scans. Predictor concepts. Supervised learning. Latent variables, topical models, causal models and time series. Object tracking and motion analysis	X-ray or thermal images are fed to the algorithm with the aim of detecting Covid-19 infection. The algorithm can be run live on the website or on a desktop, laptop or mobile embedded hardware to process images that can be deployed anywhere	Detection of sick people

Identification			Expression of need		Application of AI		Performance and purpose	
Industry/ company	Country	Expectation of the solution	Expression of the identified need	Proposed solution	Field and/or means of application of AI	Possible techniques and/or actions	Alerts and/or features	Service rendered in the therapeutic follow-up of the disease
Blockgemini	United Arab Emirates	Quarantine tracking system	This system is used to track the location of everyone who has been quarantined to ensure that they remain in their designated location at all times and avoid spreading Covid-19. This will help ensure that medical teams focus on the patients who need it	The user will receive a wrist tag which will then be synchronized with a mobile application. The user provides the location in which they will quarantine themselves, which is programmed into the application	Machine learning. Signal processing	Understanding. Deep learning trained on a set of existing CT scans. Predictor concepts. Supervised learning. Latent variables, topical models, causal models and time series. Object tracking and motion analysis	If the user leaves this location, the user and the authorities are alerted via the application and a central dashboard. The authorities can then act accordingly	Monitoring of physiological parameters

Identification			Expression of need		Application of AI		Performance and purpose	
Industry/ company	Country	Expectation of the solution	Expression of the identified need	Proposed solution	Field and/or means of application of AI	Possible techniques and/or actions	Alerts and/or features	Service rendered in the therapeutic follow-up of the disease
Mirai Innovation Research Institute	Japan	Autonomous robot to detect people with a fever	Identifying people with Covid-19 symptoms, such as a fever, in public places, such as shopping malls or airports; questioning people and isolating them as soon as possible to avoid spreading the virus to others	This solution consists of an autonomous robot that can be placed in a designated area (such as a shopping mall) and which monitors a people's body temperature, identifies people with a fever, approaches them and initiates a teleconference with a physician	Machine learning. Signal processing	Understanding. Deep learning trained on a set of existing CT scans. Predictor concepts. Supervised learning. Latent variables, topical models, causal models and time series. Object tracking and motion analysis	Autonomous navigation to patrol the designated area, artificial intelligence to detect people, use of a thermographic camera to monitor people's body temperature, interaction to approach a person with fever	Detection of sick people

Identification			Expression of need		Application of AI		Performance and purpose	
Industry/ company	Country	Expectation of the solution	Expression of the identified need	Proposed solution	Field and/or means of application of AI	Possible techniques and/or actions	Alerts and/or features	Service rendered in the therapeutic follow-up of the disease
UN MILLION DE BOT, SL	Spain	Chatbot with AI providing symptoms and information on Covid-19	The need to obtain answers to concrete questions about Covid-19 (limitations and fragmented nature of current information services)	A conversational chatbot available in English, French and Spanish that provides reliable information from official entities on Covid-19 is available 24/7 and is accessible via websites, Facebook, WhatsApp and Telegram	Robotics. Natural language processing. Signal processing. Multi-agent systems (agent = software) or distributed artificial intelligence	Cognition for robotics and systems. Design, perception, decision, action. Searching in an image bank. Object tracking and motion analysis. Multi-agent learning (language, platforms)	Answering citizens' frequently asked questions in real time in an automated way and avoiding false answers, with truthful information supervised by a multidisciplinary team and led by experts in the health sector, in addition to user geolocation, data analysis and updates to information on health measures	Communication of scientific advice

Identification			Expression of need		Application of AI		Performance and purpose	
Industry/ company	Country	Expectation of the solution	Expression of the identified need	Proposed solution	Field and/or means of application of AI	Possible techniques and/or actions	Alerts and/or features	Service rendered in the therapeutic follow-up of the disease
Robotics Flow	Denmark	flowbot ONE	Rapidly configuring liquid handling for DNA extraction and PCR tests	A simple and intuitive liquid-handling robot that can be used in research centers	Robotics. Natural language. processing Signal processing. Multi-agent systems (agent = software) or distributed artificial intelligence	Cognition for robotics and systems. Design, perception, decision, action. Searching in an image bank. Object tracking and motion analysis. Multi-agent learning (language, platforms)	Installed, trained up and deployed on the day of installation. No special training required for robotics programming	Detection of sick people

Identification			Expression of need		Application of AI		Performance and purpose	
Industry/ company	Country	Expectation of the solution	Expression of the identified need	Proposed solution	Field and/or means of application of AI	Possible techniques and/or actions	Alerts and/or features	Service rendered in the therapeutic follow-up of the disease
University of Oslo	Norway	MELODIC Cross-Cloud application management for the eScience application	Assessing which computational models are subject to data farming experiments to estimate the most likely parameters, whether the rate of spread of the contamination or the rate of mortality in real time, which depend on the proportion of the population actually infected without having been tested	MELODIC can help to manage data processing. applications that dynamically use cloud resources in their calculations	Natural language processing Signal processing Multi-agent systems (agent = software) or distributed artificial intelligence	Searching in an image bank. Object tracking and motion analysis. Multi-agent learning (language, platforms)	MELODIC takes a model of the application to be deployed and then acquires the cloud resources needed to run that application. During runtime, MELODIC measures the parameters of the running application and optimizes the resources and deployment to ensure that the application meets its deadline or computational goals	Detection of sick people

Identification		Expression of need			Application of AI		Performance and purpose	
Industry/ company	Country	Expectation of the solution	Expression of the identified need	Proposed solution	Field and/or means of application of AI	Possible techniques and/or actions	Alerts and/or features	Service rendered in the therapeutic follow-up of the disease
Health Technologies of the Canary Islands	Switzerland	Covid-19 rapid point-of-care breathing test	The need for rapid, cost-effective and scalable tests that can detect both asymptomatic and symptomatic individuals infected with Covid-19	The test has many advantages over the current point-of-care test. The three most important advantages are as follows: – it can detect the presence of the virus very early on, even in asymptomatic individuals; – it is a portable device that does not need a lab or a lab technician to operate, and the lab is a cloud-based AI system; – it has a built-in real-time monitoring feature, as all data analysis is performed in the cloud	Machine learning. Signal processing. Multi-agent systems (agent = software) or distributed artificial intelligence	Understanding. Deep learning trained on a set of existing CT scans. Predictor concepts. Supervised learning. Latent variables, topical models, causal models and time series. Object tracking and motion analysis	Canary's Covid Breath Test can detect the virus from breath alone: the individual simply breathes on the disposable device for 40 seconds. Breath data are captured by nano-sensors and sent to the cloud for analysis	Detection of sick people

Identification			Expression of need		Application of AI		Performance and purpose	
Industry/ company	**Country**	**Expectation of the solution**	**Expression of the identified need**	**Proposed solution**	**Field and/or means of application of AI**	**Possible techniques and/or actions**	**Alerts and/or features**	**Service rendered in the therapeutic follow-up of the disease**
Prisme.ai	France	Prisme.ai	Health services are currently overloaded and many processes can be automated	A Prisme.ai bot on a secure mobile application to inform, diagnose and share one's location	Robotics. Natural language processing. Signal processing. Multi-agent systems (agent = software) or distributed artificial intelligence	Cognition for robotics and systems. Design, perception, decision, action. Searching in an image bank. Object tracking and motion analysis. Multi-agent learning (language, platforms)	Mobile application and web view with a bot to provide information. The patient's location or an address is collected without displaying the result. Doctors can be alerted according to certain criteria (temperature > 40°C, etc.) and eventually call the patient	Supply chain management

Identification			Expression of need		Application of AI		Performance and purpose	
Industry/ company	Country	Expectation of the solution	Expression of the identified need	Proposed solution	Field and/or means of application of AI	Possible techniques and/or actions	Alerts and/or features	Service rendered in the therapeutic follow-up of the disease
logixlab	Malaysia	AI to detect Covid-19 using X-ray and patient data	The late detection of false positives has led to patients suffering critical complications, organ failure and death	AI chest X-ray detection for Covid-19. Transmits DICOM-based chest X-ray images over networks or the Internet to a centralized server. The data are processed using an artificial intelligence algorithm for chest X-ray interpretation	Automatic learning. Signal processing. Multi-agent systems (agent = software) or distributed artificial intelligence	Understanding. Deep learning trained on a set of existing CT scans. Predictor concepts. Supervised learning. Latent variables, topical models, causal models and time series. Object tracking and motion analysis	Health professionals create an account to ensure that the images are received and interpreted	Detection of sick people

Identification			Expression of need		Application of AI		Performance and purpose	
Industry/ company	Country	Expectation of the solution	Expression of the identified need	Proposed solution	Field and/or means of application of AI	Possible techniques and/or actions	Alerts and/or features	Service rendered in the therapeutic follow-up of the disease
ArkonIT Consulting UG	Germany	Predicting the severity of a disease	Only by obtaining a reliable statement about the expected severity of a person's illness (e.g., mild, severe, critical) can targeted medical measures be planned and initiated	Automated robots to predict health status based on preconfigured computational models	Robotics. Machine learning. Signal processing. Multi-agent systems (agent = software) or distributed artificial intelligence	Understanding. Deep learning trained on a set of existing CT scans. Predictor concepts. Supervised learning. Latent variables, topical models, causal models and time series. Object tracking and motion analysis	The model for calculating physiological parameters (e.g., weight, age, living conditions, diseases, etc.) generates a multidimensional individual model. This model can be compared with the individual model of a real person	Detection of sick people

Identification			Expression of need		Application of AI		Performance and purpose	
Industry/ company	Country	Expectation of the solution	Expression of the identified need	Proposed solution	Field and/or means of application of AI	Possible techniques and/or actions	Alerts and/or features	Service rendered in the therapeutic follow-up of the disease
targens GmbH	Germany	Covid-19 risk triage	The course of Covid-19 can vary greatly, from very mild to very critical for the patient. It is therefore essential to know as early as possible how the disease will progress from person to person	Predicting the course of the disease by proposing explanatory factors, i.e., the reasons for the specific course of a disease. Based on data from real Covid-19 cases, a machine learning model provides an AI risk triage for each new patient	Machine learning. Signal processing. Multi-agent systems (agent = software) or distributed artificial intelligence	Deep learning trained on a set of existing CT scans. Predictor concepts. Supervised learning. Latent variables, topical models, causal models and time series. Object tracking and motion analysis	Individual cases are assigned to different risk categories that predict the courses of different diseases. In addition, the reasons why an individual case has been assigned to a specific risk category are provided (e.g., age, previous diseases). Predicting the course of the disease saves valuable time for the patient	Detection of sick people

Identification			Expression of need		Application of AI		Performance and purpose	
Industry/ company	Country	Expectation of the solution	Expression of the identified need	Proposed solution	Field and/or means of application of AI	Possible techniques and/or actions	Alerts and/or features	Service rendered in the therapeutic follow-up of the disease
targens GmbH	Germany	targens conversational AI	All parts of the health-care system are currently experiencing an increase in telephone and e-mail inquiries by several orders of magnitude	The solution provides conversational AI that can handle this task in real time, 24/7. In addition, it is designed to run very efficiently on-premises or in a private cloud. No external API required	Machine learning. Signal processing. Multi-agent systems (agent = software) or distributed artificial intelligence	Deep learning that will be trained on a set of existing CT scans. Predictor concepts. Supervised learning. Latent variables, topical models, causal models and time series. Object tracking and motion analysis	The solution identifies the intention of the requester. It automatically routes the email to the appropriate recipient. It can automatically respond to simple requests. It can identify spam or make suggestions to reach the appropriate recipient if it is outside the recipient's current care organization	Communication of scientific advice

Identification			Expression of need		Application of AI		Performance and purpose	
Industry/ company	**Country**	**Expectation of the solution**	**Expression of the identified need**	**Proposed solution**	**Field and/or means of application of AI**	**Possible techniques and/or actions**	**Alerts and/or features**	**Service rendered in the therapeutic follow-up of the disease**
DMLAB	Hungary	Monitoring social distance in European cities	Ascertaining the level of social distancing in European cities. Measuring changes in foot traffic levels. Measuring the effects of governmental measures to prevent the spread of Covid-19. Ascertaining what European cities and governments can learn from each other	Foot traffic levels are calculated as percentages of normal traffic based on the daily maximum of Waze users in each city. Figures are from wazestatcom	Multi-agent systems (agent = software) or distributed artificial intelligence. Machine learning	Deep learning. Supervised learning. Latent variables, topical models, causal models and time series	Foot traffic levels are used as indicators of social distancing in cities. The second section of the dashboard maps actual government actions to the timing of traffic changes	Assessment of social distancing

Identification			Expression of need		Application of AI		Performance and purpose	
Industry/ company	Country	Expectation of the solution	Expression of the identified need	Proposed solution	Field and/or means of application of AI	Possible techniques and/or actions	Alerts and/or features	Service rendered in the therapeutic follow-up of the disease
Sensifai	Belgium	Automatic detection of Covid-19 in radiographic and CT images	Numerous studies show that Covid-19 causes specific abnormalities in chest X-ray images. Although X-ray imaging is available to most people, consulting specialists to interpret X-ray images is too costly and time consuming, and even impossible due to the overwhelming number of suspected patients	Sensifai technology enables the detection of Covid-19 patients through X-ray images of the lungs	Multi-agent systems (agent = software) or distributed artificial intelligence. Machine learning. Signal processing	Deep learning with cloud-based microprocessors to recognize Covid-19 patients while ensuring their privacy. Supervised learning. Latent variables, topical models, causal models and time series	An artificial intelligence solution that automatically analyzes X-rays in less than a second and detects Covid-19 patients	Detection of sick people

Identification			Expression of need		Application of AI		Performance and purpose	
Industry/ company	**Country**	**Expectation of the solution**	**Expression of the identified need**	**Proposed solution**	**Field and/or means of application of AI**	**Possible techniques and/or actions**	**Alerts and/or features**	**Service rendered in the therapeutic follow-up of the disease**
RAYLYTIC GmbH	Germany	UNITY: a medical research and crisis management platform	Digital monitoring of research data	UNITY is a web-based clinical trial management platform. With its hierarchical data and information model, it allows for central deployment on a national scale, combining local triage and information needs	Multi-agent systems (agent = software) or distributed artificial intelligence	Multi-agent learning. Distributed problem solving	Patient triage. Real-world granular data collection to assess risks and benefits and obtain real-time status information. Manages knowledge distribution and data collection needs with local patient information and workflows	Communication of scientific advice

Identification			Expression of need		Application of AI		Performance and purpose	
Industry/ company	Country	Expectation of the solution	Expression of the identified need	Proposed solution	Field and/or means of application of AI	Possible techniques and/or actions	Alerts and/or features	Service rendered in the therapeutic follow-up of the disease
Black Swan Lux	Luxembourg	SafeLive application	Tracking a person's path (location) and monitoring a range of biometric parameters. Automatically detecting anomalies, such as people deviating from their usual routine, in terms of location, daily rhythm, biometric parameters, etc.	Real-time tracking and health monitoring via devices such as smart watches. Automatic alerts triggered by AI/ML in case of anomalies, such as unusual location, heart rate, activity, etc. The solution builds a profile of the person wearing the watch and learns in near real time	N/A	/	In an emergency, the wearer can also trigger an alert that is received by health-care providers or people nearby via a mobile application. Mapping the network of interactions of users to identify people at risk based on past encounters	Monitoring of physiological parameters

Identification			Expression of need		Application of AI		Performance and purpose	
Industry/ company	Country	Expectation of the solution	Expression of the identified need	Proposed solution	Field and/or means of application of AI	Possible techniques and/or actions	Alerts and/or features	Service rendered in the therapeutic follow-up of the disease
OESIA NETWORKS	Spain	Biometric data analysis platform	The need to analyze all types of structured medical and biological data, resource data and logistics data to obtain predictions on any type of target for medical and resource planning purposes to deal with a pandemic	Artificial intelligence platform running in a computer capable of executing more than 200 supervised and unsupervised mathematical models developed after 13 years of fundamental research	Multi-agent systems (agent = software) or distributed artificial intelligence	Multi-agent learning. Distributed problem solving	Biological databases, vaccine simulation, mass sequencing, gene comparison in Open Source	Prediction of disease progression

Identification			Expression of need		Application of AI		Performance and purpose	
Industry/ company	**Country**	**Expectation of the solution**	**Expression of the identified need**	**Proposed solution**	**Field and/or means of application of AI**	**Possible techniques and/or actions**	**Alerts and/or features**	**Service rendered in the therapeutic follow-up of the disease**
HealthBeats	Singapore	HealthBeats remote vital data monitoring solution	Remote vital signs monitoring can be deployed to monitor patients' vital signs, such as temperature, oxygen level, blood pressure, etc. This reduces the workload and improves the efficiency of health-care professionals	A remote vital monitoring platform designed to bring healthcare to the home with a focus on each healthcare user's experience (providers and patients). The patient can easily take measurements at home	Multi-agent systems (agent = software) or distributed artificial intelligence	Multi-agent learning. Distributed problem solving	The HealthBeats solution involves providing users with medical devices to self-administer on a regular basis at home and transmitting their results in real time to healthcare providers for proactive care management	Monitoring of physiological parameters

Identification			Expression of need		Application of AI		Performance and purpose	
Industry/ company	Country	Expectation of the solution	Expression of the identified need	Proposed solution	Field and/or means of application of AI	Possible techniques and/or actions	Alerts and/or features	Service rendered in the therapeutic follow-up of the disease
Spa Expert System	Italy	Medical Information Platform: MIP	The product was designed to improve the public's ability to understand the methodologies, operational capabilities, modus operandi and techniques used by state and non-state actors against various types of attacks and risks, adopting the Health Intelligence paradigm to digitally track the emergence of new outbreaks and the chain of infection	Platform for managing megadata correlated to the coronavirus pandemic, providing a horizontal scanning system to detect low indicators and weak signals	Machine learning. Signal processing. Multi-agent systems (agent = software) or distributed artificial intelligence	Deep learning trained on a set of existing CT scans. Predictor concepts. Supervised learning. Latent variables, topical models, causal models and time series. Object tracking and motion analysis	Quickly identifies relevant correlations between data from different sources (open sources and other medical sources) and supports tactical and strategic decisions	Communication of scientific advice

Identification			Expression of need		Application of AI		Performance and purpose	
Industry/ company	**Country**	**Expectation of the solution**	**Expression of the identified need**	**Proposed solution**	**Field and/or means of application of AI**	**Possible techniques and/or actions**	**Alerts and/or features**	**Service rendered in the therapeutic follow-up of the disease**
Consortium: EusoMII.org, Robovision.eu, NK.Inl and Quibim.com	Belgium	Automated diagnosis and analysis of Covid-19 based on CT scans	Analyzing and quantifying abnormalities in CT images performed with patients with a suspected Covid-19 infection and prioritizing individual cases to save lives at critical times when the workflow is extremely high and human effort requires considerable focus	An artificial intelligence solution to collect CT images of lungs from patients. This is performed according to a multi-center scientific research protocol	Machine learning. Signal processing. Multi-agent systems (agent = software) or distributed artificial intelligence	Deep learning trained on a set of existing CT scans. Predictor concepts. Supervised learning. Latent variables, topical models, causal models and time series. Object tracking and motion analysis	The images are collected, prepared and used for scientific research	Detection of sick people

Identification			Expression of need		Application of AI		Performance and purpose	
Industry/ company	Country	Expectation of the solution	Expression of the identified need	Proposed solution	Field and/or means of application of AI	Possible techniques and/or actions	Alerts and/or features	Service rendered in the therapeutic follow-up of the disease
Site-Kicks	Netherlands	Questions and answers about Covid-19	Academic research is produced in very large volumes. Moreover, new publications come out so fast that it is almost impossible to read them and filter out reliable information	Using all academic articles to form a knowledge base where you can ask questions that appear as clear answers	Machine learning	Deep learning that will be trained on a set of existing CT scans. Predictor concepts	Covid-19 knowledge base	Communication of scientific advice
Neuroteg AI	Belgium	Zero contact Covid-19 robot	With a humanoid robot, a person's temperature, oxygen saturation, respiratory rate, HR and HRV can be detected	A robot with an integrated camera that provides transdermal optical imaging	Robotics. Natural language processing. Signal processing. Multi-agent systems (agent = software) or distributed artificial intelligence	Cognition for robotics and systems. Design, perception, decision, action. Searching in an image bank. Object tracking and motion analysis. Multi-agent learning (language, platforms)	/	Detection of sick people

Identification			Expression of need		Application of AI		Performance and purpose	
Industry/ company	Country	Expectation of the solution	Expression of the identified need	Proposed solution	Field and/or means of application of AI	Possible techniques and/or actions	Alerts and/or features	Service rendered in the therapeutic follow-up of the disease
Unacast	Norway	Social distancing dashboard by Unacast	What is known is that the virus is more contagious than the flu and that social distancing seems to be an effective way to slow its spread and thus give health services the opportunity to deal with the increased number of people needing emergency care and save lives	Real World Graph®, a suite of products based on geospatial information on human mobility. New models based on real-time data to accurately measure the effectiveness of different social distancing strategies in the real world	Multi-agent systems (agent = software) or distributed artificial intelligence	Multi-agent learning. Distributed problem solving	Helping the government, states, counties and cities take the best action on social distancing using a social distancing dashboard and dataset	Communication of scientific advice

Identification			Expression of need		Application of AI		Performance and purpose	
Industry/ company	Country	Expectation of the solution	Expression of the identified need	Proposed solution	Field and/or means of application of AI	Possible techniques and/or actions	Alerts and/or features	Service rendered in the therapeutic follow-up of the disease
Yourmd	United Kingdom	YourMD	People with non-Covid symptoms can be helped and asymptomatic people can be detected, traced and put into isolation	a) Help people assess themselves appropriately for Covid-19; (b) development of a Covid-19 self-assessment tool; (c) a coronavirus information center; (d) daily isolation with news and tips for surviving the lockdown by looking at food, sleep, activit, and mental health; (e) symptom tracking for people with mild, moderate and severe symptoms; (f) a 14-day quarantine partner to help people manage their isolation with the virus	/	/	Disinfection and sterilization	Disinfection

Identification			Expression of need		Application of AI		Performance and purpose	
Industry/ company	Country	Expectation of the solution	Expression of the identified need	Proposed solution	Field and/or means of application of AI	Possible techniques and/or actions	Alerts and/or features	Service rendered in the therapeutic follow-up of the disease
Kanteron Systems SLU	Spain	Kanteron platform for Covid-19	Prevention, diagnostic accuracy, geographic coverage and real-time reporting	Allows some health workers to work remotely (teleradiology, telepathology, telegenomics), avoiding contagion and the unnecessary reduction of required health staff. Uses one or more diagnostic methods (PCR, US, XRays, CT, WSI, etc.) and integrates the results with the patient EMR. Care (from diagnosis to treatment and follow-up) can be provided remotely, maximizing both geographic coverage and the availability of limited resources. Real-time population health and epidemiology reporting	/	/	Healthcare professionals remotely create their account in 10 minutes and send the link/SMS to their existing or potential patient households. Patients can communicate to provide information about their health. Sharing languages available: English, Italian, Spanish, German and French	Telemedicine

Identification			Expression of need		Application of AI		Performance and purpose	
Industry/ company	**Country**	**Expectation of the solution**	**Expression of the identified need**	**Proposed solution**	**Field and/or means of application of AI**	**Possible techniques and/or actions**	**Alerts and/or features**	**Service rendered in the therapeutic follow-up of the disease**
Coventry University	United Kingdom	Machine–clinician–hybrid intelligence for Covid-19 diagnosis	A rapid test for the virus is clinically and socially important. Viral nucleic acid detection is the common method but suffers from low efficiency and high false-negative rates. Chest CT screening has been used as the main complementary tool in China and other epidemic areas to stratify risk in patients. Unfortunately, clinicians' analyses of CT images require a great deal of expertise and are time-consuming, so an automated alternative is urgently needed to obtain a rapid diagnosis	Through collaborations between experienced AI researchers (at Coventry University), clinicians/radiologists and an AI MedTech SME (in China) based on a new AI solution for Covid-19, this solution combines the power of deep learning models and the domain expertise of the clinician to make an effective, reliable and explainable diagnosis, evaluate it specifically for the EU population and then explore the best implementation strategy for the EU healthcare system	/	/	Disinfection and sterilization	Disinfection

Identification			Expression of need		Application of AI		Performance and purpose	
Industry/ company	**Country**	**Expectation of the solution**	**Expression of the identified need**	**Proposed solution**	**Field and/or means of application of AI**	**Possible techniques and/or actions**	**Alerts and/or features**	**Service rendered in the therapeutic follow-up of the disease**
Mes modèles de données	France	TADA, a machine learning platform for health research	Covid-19 researchers are under pressure to analyze disease behavior and its impact on patient health. New data and new hypotheses are coming in daily. Results have a significant effect on how countries respond to the pandemic	The Mes modèles de données (My Data Models) product uses the latest advances in artificial intelligence to build interpretable models of the data. By reviewing these models, researchers can find patterns and discover new correlations that would have taken days to find using traditional methods. The solution is currently used in healthcare on a daily basis to diagnose cancers and propose drugs to patients with rare diseases. Concerning Covid-19, we have confirmed with researchers in France that the tool can help	Machine learning	/	Healthcare professionals remotely create their account in 10 minutes and send the link/SMS to their existing or potential patient households. Patients can communicate to provide information about their health. Sharing languages available: English, Italian, Spanish, German and French	Medical research on a treatment

Identification			Expression of need		Application of AI		Performance and purpose	
Industry/ company	Country	Expectation of the solution	Expression of the identified need	Proposed solution	Field and/or means of application of AI	Possible techniques and/or actions	Alerts and/or features	Service rendered in the therapeutic follow-up of the disease
Octinion	Belgium	Autonomous UVC vehicle to disinfect corridors	On account of Covid-19, continuous cleaning is required. This requires a lot of effort and therefore the focus is on the most critical areas such as surgery, restrooms and patient rooms. However, there are many other areas, such as corridors, that are also a potential risk and where most of the time only the floor is cleaned. Our solution is specifically adapted to disinfect surfaces such as walls, doors and other visible objects in corridors and halls	UVC light can kill the coronavirus. A dose of 12 J/m^2 is already sufficient to kill it with 97% certainty. A vehicle is equipped with UVC lamps and driven at 3 km/h to provide the 12 J/m dose. By lowering the speed, the dose can be increased. The vehicle operates autonomously so that cleaning personnel can continue to focus on the most critical areas	/	/	Disinfection and sterilization	Disinfection

Identification			Expression of need		Application of AI		Performance and purpose	
Industry/ company	Country	Expectation of the solution	Expression of the identified need	Proposed solution	Field and/or means of application of AI	Possible techniques and/or actions	Alerts and/or features	Service rendered in the therapeutic follow-up of the disease
BioRICS NV	Belgium	Infection detection, accessible in in real time	The problem is the ability to detect a viral infection at an early stage. People working in the healthcare sector are at greater risk of infection than people working in other sectors. Once infected, these workers must be immediately removed from the workplace to prevent them from infecting others. However, Covid testing is time consuming and not sufficiently available. There is therefore a strong need for accessible testing based on ongoing surveillance	BioRICS' Mindstretch solution measures key variables in real time according to a human's individual metabolic energy equation. Using a wearable device, such as a Fitbit, combined with individualized AI-based algorithms, the energy the body consumes for multiple tasks is calculated. Mindstretch's next-generation algorithms have proven successful in detecting small-scale infections as they are caused by the Covid-19 virus. The algorithms provide their information via a web portal or smartphone application	/	/	Healthcare professionals remotely create their account in 10 minutes and send the link/SMS to their existing or potential patient households. Patients can communicate to provide information about their health. Sharing languages available: English, Italian, Spanish, German and French	Detection of sick people

Identification			Expression of need		Application of AI		Performance and purpose	
Industry/ company	Country	Expectation of the solution	Expression of the identified need	Proposed solution	Field and/or means of application of AI	Possible techniques and/or actions	Alerts and/or features	Service rendered in the therapeutic follow-up of the disease
À domicile	Belgium	Soline	Interaction between Covid-19 patients and nurses: Soline enables the patient to interact without physical contact with the hospital/institution staff by initiating a phone call or nurse call via voice, gesture or sight. Interaction between Covid-19 patients and hospital room equipment: as for the nurse call, the use of the television, the telephone, the positioning of the bed, the lights, the blinds and the door can be controlled in a contactless way or using an adapted interaction mode	Soline is a platform that enables the control of features with over ten different modes of interaction. Basic features include nurse calls, telephone, television, music, audio books and radio. Control of the bed, lights, fixtures and door are optional features. Possible interaction modes are voice, gesture, sight, touch devices, switches, remote controls, wheelchair joystick, communication software, push buttons, mice, etc.	/	/	Disinfection and sterilization	Disinfection

Identification			Expression of need		Application of AI		Performance and purpose	
Industry/ company	Country	Expectation of the solution	Expression of the identified need	Proposed solution	Field and/or means of application of AI	Possible techniques and/or actions	Alerts and/or features	Service rendered in the therapeutic follow-up of the disease
Enversion	Denmark	+ PrioAcute	Waiting times have a significant impact on patient mortality, readmission, resuscitation, length of stay, patient satisfaction and costs. Patient prioritization is therefore critical in the emergency department, and during a pandemic, the need for proper prioritization is crucial for citizens and clinicians	+ PrioAcute helps clinical staff prioritize patients by separating high-risk from low-risk patients in the visitation process. Today, the visitation process lacks historical information about the patient, making it difficult to predict the patient's future course. + PrioAcute uses this information along with new acute disease information to improve this prediction through artificial intelligence	/	/	Healthcare professionals remotely create their account in 10 minutes and send the link/SMS to their existing or potential patient households. Patients can communicate to provide information about their health. Sharing languages available: English, Italian, Spanish, German and French	Monitoring of physiological parameters

Identification			Expression of need		Application of AI		Performance and purpose	
Industry/ company	Country	Expectation of the solution	Expression of the identified need	Proposed solution	Field and/or means of application of AI	Possible techniques and/or actions	Alerts and/or features	Service rendered in the therapeutic follow-up of the disease
IMMUNOSTEP SL	Spain	Robotic platform for Covid-19 cytometry studies (Cytoprep)	The patient's response, as well as possible treatments and clinical management, depend on the state of their immune system. In this sense, in order to undertake this study at the clinical level, flow cytometry plays an important role, but the preparation of the samples is usually done manually due to the large number of reagents used. However, in the case of Covid-19-positive samples, the preparation may compromise the safety of the laboratory technicians	A robotic platform for the preparation of samples for flow cytometry that fits into a type II A2 biological safety cabinet, for the P3 containment level	/	/	Disinfection and sterilization	Disinfection

Identification			Expression of need		Application of AI		Performance and purpose	
Industry/ company	**Country**	**Expectation of the solution**	**Expression of the identified need**	**Proposed solution**	**Field and/or means of application of AI**	**Possible techniques and/or actions**	**Alerts and/or features**	**Service rendered in the therapeutic follow-up of the disease**
Jozef Stefan Institute	Slovenia	Coronavirus Watch portal: multimedia and analytical visualizations	AI analysis methods used to track media and visualize the spread of Covid-19 across the world and countries	The solution uses semantic and multilingual processing to collect/process/ visualize media, and advanced analytical visualization techniques to present the spread of the coronavirus worldwide and by country	/	/	Healthcare professionals remotely create their account in 10 minutes and send the link/SMS to their existing or potential patient households. Patients can communicate to provide information about their health. Sharing languages available: English, Italian, Spanish, German and French	Prediction of disease progression

Identification			Expression of need		Application of AI		Performance and purpose	
Industry/ company	**Country**	**Expectation of the solution**	**Expression of the identified need**	**Proposed solution**	**Field and/or means of application of AI**	**Possible techniques and/or actions**	**Alerts and/or features**	**Service rendered in the therapeutic follow-up of the disease**
Dirigeable	Italy	Beat Covid-19 (BC19)	Applying social distancing measures and detecting highly vulnerable individuals in public spaces (i.e., hospitals, clinics, train stations, airports), commercial activities (i.e., supermarkets, pharmacies), and production facilities	The BC19 solution provides real-time notifications of social distancing violations and the presence of highly vulnerable individuals to facilitate data-driven actions to maximize personal and employee safety. The solution consists of a privacy-compliant smart sensor to automatically detect and alert end users about risky situations and vulnerable individuals and a cloud platform to visualize data and manage alerts	/	/	Disinfection and sterilization	Prediction of disease progression

Glossary

Acute illness: An alteration in the general state of health. It is characterized by identified symptoms, progression and recovery.

Chronic disease: Unlike an acute illness, chronic disease evolves over a long period of time and tends to get progressively worse. Its evolution is marked by acute events called relapses. These long-term diseases cannot usually be prevented by a vaccine or completely cured.

Congenital disease: A disease or malformation present at birth. Congenital diseases can be due to genetic abnormalities, the intrauterine environment or unknown factors.

Contagion: The spread of an infectious disease between individuals of the same population. Contagion by direct transmission occurs from an individual carrying the pathogen (possibly a healthy carrier) to a healthy individual. When transmission is indirect, for example through a mosquito, as in the case of malaria, it is not a contagious disease.

Contagiousness: Contagiousness refers to the potential for transmission of a contagious disease from one individual to another. The contaminated patient can contaminate a greater or lesser number depending on the type of pathogen.

Containment: A word used in a specific sense in many fields. In the health field, containment is part of a set of sanitary measures called "barrier measures", such as mask wearing for contaminated people or frequent handwashing for everyone, designed to limit the spread of a pathogen.

Contamination: Contamination refers to the fact that an individual is infected by a pathogen.

Fatality: Fatality expresses the number of deaths in the proportion of the population affected by a disease.

Hereditary disease: A disease transmitted to an individual in their genes. The disease is inherited from the parents. The disease can be dominant (i.e. occurring in every generation) or recessive (i.e. occurring from time to time).

Incubation period: The time between infection and the appearance of the first symptoms of the disease. For instance, the incubation period for influenza is 1–3 days, while for Covid-19, it is 2–14 days.

Integrated political crisis response (IPCR): A mechanism for a political reaction in a crisis situation.

Lockdown: The process of forcing a person to stay at home for a set period of time to avoid infecting others.

Mortality: The number of deaths caused by a disease in a given population over a given period of time.

The three epidemic stages of Covid-19: These are not epidemiological stages in the medical sense of the term but political decisions taken at a national level:

– stage 1 aims to slow down the introduction of the virus into a country, notably by imposing "quarantine" measures on people returning from high-risk areas, in particular the Chinese province of Hubei, where the epidemic started;

– stage 2 aims to prevent the spread of the disease. It consists of identifying the areas of virus circulation in which so-called "cluster" cases are multiplying and applying restrictive measures to these areas;

– stage 3 aims to manage the consequences of the epidemic as best as possible and to mitigate its harmful effects. This stage is characterized by the circulation of the virus within an entire territory, by which point it is much too late to enforce lockdown measures.

References

Alpay, L.L., Henkemans, O.B., Otten, W., Rövekamp, T.A.J.M., Dumay, A.C.M. (2010). E-health applications and services for patient empowerment: Directions for best practices in The Netherlands. *Tele-med. J. E. Health*, 16(7), 787–791 [Online]. Available at: https://www.liebertpub.com/doi/10.1089/tmj.2009.0156.

Aneja, S., Chang, E., Omuro, A. (2019). Applications of artificial intelligence in neurooncology. *Current Opinion in Neurology*, 32(6), 850–856.

Arbib, M.A. (1975). Artificial intelligence and brain theory: Unities and diversities. *Annals of Biomedical Engineering*, 3(3), 238–274.

Beyala, L. (2015). *Connected Objects in Health: Risks, Uses and Perspectives*. ISTE Press, London and Elsevier Ltd, Oxford.

Blei, D.M. (2012). Probabilistic topic models. *Communications of the ACM*, 55(4), 77–84.

Blumenthal, D. and Tavenner, M. (2010). The "meaningful use" regulation for electronic health records. *N. Engl. J. Med.*, 5(363), 501–504.

Body, R., Carley, S., Wibberley, C., McDowell, G., Ferguson, J., Mackway-Jones, K. (2010). The value of symptoms and signs in the emergent diagnosis of acute coronary syndromes. *Resuscitation*, 81(3), 281–286.

Body, R., Mueller, C., Giannitsis, E. (2016). The use of very low concentrations of high-sensitivity troponin T to rule out acute myocardial infarction using a single blood test. *Acad. Emerg. Med.*, 23(9), 1004–1013.

Carlton, E.W., Than, M., Cullen, L., Khattab, A., Greaves, K. (2015). "Chest pain typicality" in suspected acute coronary syndromes and the impact of clinical experience. *Am. J. Med.*, 128(10), 1109–1116.

Chen, X., Zhang, X., Xie, H., Wang, F.L., Yan, J., Hao, T. (2019). Trends and features of human brain research using artificial intelligence techniques: A bibliometric approach. In *Human Brain and Artificial Intelligence*, Zheng, A., Pan, D., Hao, T., Zhang, D., Shi, Y., Song, X. (eds). Springer Publishing, New York.

Communications Authority of Kenya (2015). First quarter sector statistics report for the financial year 2015/2016. Report, Communications Authority of Kenya, Nairobi.

Déglise, C., Suggs, L.S., Odermatt, P. (2012). SMS for disease control in developing countries: A systematic review of mobile health applications. *J. Telemed. Telecare*, 18(5), 273–281.

Du, H.S., Ke, X., Chu, S.K., Chan, L.T. (2017). A bibliometric analysis of emergency management using information systems (2000–2016). *Online Information Review*, 41(4), 454–470.

Garfield, E. (1964). "Science citation index" – A new dimension in indexing. *Science*, 144(3619), 649–654.

Geng, Y., Chen, W., Liu, Z., Chiu, A.S., Han, W., Liu, Z., Zhong, S., Qian, Y., You, W., Cui, X. (2017). A bibliometric review: Energy consumption and greenhouse gas emissions in the residential sector. *Journal of Cleaner Production*, 159, 301–316.

Ghebreab, S. (2021). Fighting inequality with the help of artificial intelligence [Online]. Available at: https://www.uva.nl/en/shared-content/faculteiten/en/faculteit-der-natuurwetenschappen-wiskunde-en-informatica/news/2021/06/sennay-ghebreab-jaaroverzicht-2020.html?cb&cb.

Graham, S., Depp, C., Lee, E.E., Nebeker, C., Tu, X., Kim, H.-C., Jeste, D.V. (2019). Artificial intelligence for mental health and mental illnesses: An overview. *Current Psychiatry Reports*, 21(11), 116.

Greenhalgh, T. and Keen, J. (2013). England's national programme for IT [Online]. Available at: https://www.bmj.com/content/346/bmj.f4130/rr/653674. *BMJ*, 346.

Greenslade, J.H., Cullen, L., Parsonage, W. (2012). Examining the signs and symptoms experienced by individuals with suspected acute coronary syndrome in the Asia-Pacific region: A prospective observational study. *Ann. Emerg. Med.*, 60(6), 777–785.

Hassabis, D., Kumaran, D., Summerfield, C., Botvinick, M. (2017). Neuroscience-inspired artificial intelligence. *Neuron*, 95(2), 245–258.

Hassan, S.-U., Haddawy, P., Zhu, J. (2014). A bibliometric study of the world's research activity in sustainable development and its sub-areas using scientific literature. *Scientometrics*, 99, 549–574.

Hess, E.P., Agarwal, D., Chandra, S. (2010). Diagnostic accuracy of the TIMI risk score in patients with chest pain in the emergency department: A meta-analysis. *Can. Med. Assoc. J.*, 182(10), 1039–1044.

Jiang, H., Qiang, M., Lin, P.A. (2016). A topic modeling-based bibliometric exploration of hydropower research. *Renewable and Sustainable Energy*, 57, 226–237.

Jiang, H., Qiang, M., Fan, Q., Zhang, M. (2018). Scientific research driven by large-scale infrastructure projects: A case study of the Three Gorges Project in China. *Technological Forecasting and Social Change*, 134, 61–71.

Kamal, H., Lopez, V., Sheth, S.A. (2018). Machine learning in acute ischemic stroke neuroimaging. *Frontiers in Neurology*, 8(9), 945.

Kuperman, G.J. (2011). Health-information exchange: Why are we doing it, and what are we doing? *J. Am. Med. Inform. Assoc.*, 18(5), 678–682.

Lee, E.-J., Kim, Y.-H., Kim, N., Kang, D.-W. (2017). Deep into the brain: Artificial intelligence in stroke imaging. *Journal of Stroke*, 19(3), 277–285.

Lewis, T., Synowiec, C., Lagomarsino, G., Schweitzer, J. (2012). E-health in low- and middle-income countries: Findings from the Center for Health Market Innovations. *Bull. World Health Organ.*, 90(5), 334–340.

Mahler, S.A., Miller, C.D., Hollander, J.E. (2013). Identifying patients for early discharge: Performance of decision rules among patients with acute chest pain. *Int. J. Cardiol.*, 168(2), 795–802.

National Statistics (2015). Hospital episode statistics, admitted patient care. Report, Department of Health, London.

Obasola, O.I., Mabawonku, I., Lagunju, I. (2015). A review of e-health interventions for maternal and child health in sub-Sahara Africa. *Matern. Child Health J.*, 19, 1813–1824.

Sakai, K. and Yamada, K. (2019). Machine learning studies on major brain diseases: 5-year trends of 2014–2018. *Japanese Journal of Radiology*, 37(1), 34–72.

Senders, J.T., Staples, P.C., Karhade, A.V., Zaki, M.M., Gormley, W.B., Broekman, M.L., Smith, T.R., Arnaout, O. (2018a). Machine learning and neurosurgical outcome prediction: A systematic review. *World Neurosurgery*, 109, 476–486.

Senders, J.T., Zaki, M.M., Karhade, A.V., Chang, B., Gormley, W.B, Broekman, M.L., Smith, T.R., Arnaout, O. (2018b). An introduction and overview of machine learning in neurosurgical care. *Acta Neurochirurgica*, 160(1), 29–38.

Shaver, M., Kohanteb, P., Chiou, C., Bardis, M.D., Chantaduly, C., Bota, D., Filippi, C.G., Weinberg, B., Grinband, J., Chow, D.S., Chang, P.D. (2019). Optimizing neuro-oncology imaging: A review of deep learning approaches for glioma imaging. *Cancers*, 11(6), 829.

Than, M.P., Pickering, J.W., Aldous, S.J. (2016). Effectiveness of EDACS versus ADAPT accelerated diagnostic pathways for chest pain: A pragmatic randomized controlled trial embedded within practice. *Ann. Emerg. Med.*, 68(1), 93–102.

Tierney, W.M., Achieng, M., Baker, E., Bell, A., Biondich, P., Braitstein, P., Kayiwa, D., Kimaiyo, S., Mamlin, B., McKown, B. (2010). Experience implementing electronic health records in three East African countries. *Stud. Health Technol. Inform.*, 160, 371–375.

Tomlinson, M., Rotheram-Borus, M.J., Swartz, L., Tsai, A.C. (2013). Scaling up mHealth: Where is the evidence? *PLoS Med.*, 10(2) [Online]. Available at: https://pubmed.ncbi.nlm.nih.gov/23424286/.

Ullman, S. (1986). Artificial intelligence and the brain: Computational studies of the visual system. *Annual Review of Neuroscience*, 9, 1–26.

Ullman, S. (2019). Using neuroscience to develop artificial intelligence. *Science*, 363(6428), 692–693.

Van Gemert-Pijnen, J.E., Nijland, N., van Limburg, M., Ossebaard, H.C., Kelders, S.M., Eysenbach, G., Seydel, E.R. (2011). A holistic framework to improve the uptake and impact of e-health technologies. *J. Med. Internet Res.*, 5(13), 111.

Weiner, J.P., Yeh, S., Blumenthal, D. (2013). The impact of health information technology and e-health on the future demand for physician services. *Health Aff. (Millwood)*, 32(11), 1998–2004.

Xu, J. and Zhang, M. (2019). Use of magnetic resonance imaging and artificial intelligence in studies of diagnosis of Parkinson's disease. *ACS Chemical Neuroscience*, 10(6), 2658–2667.

Websites

https://www.aquaportail.com/definition-4437-ecosysteme-aquatique.html

https://archipel.uqam.ca/3960/1/M11905.pdf: Facteurs d'acceptation et d'utilisation des technologies d'information : une étude empirique sur l'usage du logiciel Rational Suite par les employés d'une grande compagnie de services informatiques.

https://www.cairn.info/revue-anthropologie-des-connaissances-2019-1-page-279.htm

https://www.consilium.europa.eu/fr/policies/ipcr-response-to-crises/

https://corpus.ulaval.ca/jspui/bitstream/20.500.11794/28256/1/33744.pdf

https://www.digitalcorsaire.com/formes-innovations

https://ec.europa.eu/digital-single-market/en/news/white-paper-artificial-intelligence-public-consultation-towards-european-approach-excellence

https://www.europarl.europa.eu/doceo/document/TA-9-2020-10-05-TOC_EN.html

https://www.europarl.europa.eu/news/en/press-room/20200615IPR81228/parliament-sets-up-special-committees-and-a-permanent-subcommittee

https://www.europarl.europa.eu/plenary/en/texts-adopted.html

https://www.fondationdelavenir.org/wp-content/uploads/2015/11/2015_petitguide_sante_numerique.pdf

https://www.fortunebusinessinsights.com/dental-impression-tray-market-103335

https://en.wikipedia.org/wiki/SARS

https://ici.radio-canada.ca/nouvelle/1705879/industrie-pharmaceutique-prix-baisse-reglement-delai-pandemie

https://ici.radio-canada.ca/nouvelle/1289996/medicaments-brevets-reglement-compagnies-pharmaceutiques-cout

https://www.lesechos.fr/monde/europe/litalie-place-15-millions-dhabitants-en-quarantaine-1183012

https://www.lemoniteurdespharmacies.fr

https://www.letemps.ch/monde/loms-qualifie-desormais-lepidemie-covid19-pandemie-nouvelles-11-mars

https://www.macsf.fr/responsabilite-professionnelle/cadre-juridique/telesoin-une-pratique-qui-devient-perenne-pour-les-paramedicaux-et-les-pharmaciens: Tout savoir sur le télésoin – MACSF

https://news.un.org/fr/story/2020/01/1060551: Nouveau coronavirus : premiers cas signalés en Europe (OMS) – ONU Info https://www.nutripro.nestle.fr/article/maladie-chronique-outils-connectes: Maladies chroniques, Internet et outils connectés : quel impact ?

https://www.oecd-ilibrary.org/docserver/9789264060289-11-fr.pdf?expires=1609346976&id=id&accname=guest&checksum=1DE7207A52CAE68FDEFB3EA2F54518BD

https://www.ouest-france.fr/sante/virus/coronavirus/coronavirus-quelles-sont-les-mesures-prises-en-europe-pour-eviter-la-propagation-du-virus-6778616

http://www.sietmanagement.fr/utaut/: UTAUT, TAM 3, Modèles unifiés d'acceptation des technologies – V. Venkatesh

https://www.vocabulaire-medical.fr/encyclopedie/141-endemie-epidemie-epidemiologie-pandemie#:~:text=Maladies%20%2F%20Patients%20%2F%20Pathologie-,Les%20trois%20termes%20%C2%AB%20end%C3%A9mie%20%C2%BB%2C%20%C2%AB%20%C3%A9pid%C3%A9mie%20%C2%BB%20et%20%C2%AB,parfois%20transmissibles%20%C3%A0%20l'homme

https://www.vie-publique.fr/catalogue/23844-lunion-europeenne-institutions-et-politiques

https://www.vie-publique.fr/en-bref/273953-coronavirus-fermeture-des-frontieres-de-lue-et-soutien-economique

https://webhelp.com/fr/le-groupe/

https://en.wikipedia.org/wiki/Outsourcing#Nearshoring

Index

S, T, U, W

Other titles from

ISTE

in

Health Engineering and Society

2022

ASSAILLY Jean-Pascal
Child Psychology: Developments in Knowledge and Theoretical Models
(Health and Patients Set – Volume 3)

CHAABANE Sondès, COUSEIN Etienne, WIESER Philippe
Healthcare Systems: Challenges and Opportunities

PAGANELLI Céline, CLAVIER Viviane
Information Practices and Knowledge in Health
(Health and Patients Set – Volume 5)

SALGUES Bruno, BARNOUIN Jacques
The Covid-19 Crisis: From a Question of an Epidemic to a Societal Questioning
(Health and Patients Set - Volume 4)

2021

BÉRANGER Jérôme
Societal Responsibility of Artificial Intelligence: Towards an Ethical and Eco-responsible AI
(Technological Prospects and Social Applications Set – Volume 4)

CORDELIER Benoit, GALIBERT Olivier
Digital Health Communications
(Technological Prospects and Social Applications Set – Volume 5)

NADOT Michel
Discipline of Nursing: Three-time Knowledge

2020

BARBET Jacques, FOUCQUIER Adrien, THOMAS Yves
Therapeutic Progress in Oncology: Towards a Revolution in Cancer Therapy?
(Health and Patients Set – Volume 2)

MORILLON Laurent, CLAVIER Viviane
Health Research Practices in a Digital Context
(Health Information Set – Volume 4)

PAILLIART Isabelle
New Territories in Health
(Health Information Set – Volume 3)

2019

CLAVIER Viviane, DE OLIVEIRA Jean-Philippe
Food and Health: Actor Strategies in Information and Communication
(Health Information Set – Volume 2)

PIZON Frank
Health Education and Prevention
(Health and Patients Set – Volume 1)

2018

HUARD Pierre
The Management of Chronic Diseases: Organizational Innovation and Efficiency

PAGANELLI Céline
Confidence and Legitimacy in Health Information and Communication (Health Information Set – Volume 1)

2017

PICARD Robert
Co-design in Living Labs for Healthcare and Independent Living: Concepts, Methods and Tools

2015

BÉRANGER Jérôme
Medical Information Systems Ethics

Printed and bound by CPI Group (UK) Ltd, Croydon, CR0 4YY

16/09/2026

14963075-0001